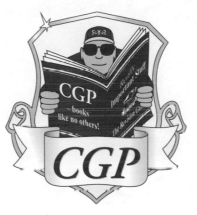

GCSE History is always topical with CGP...

"Health and the People: c1000 to the Present Day" can be a gruesome part of AQA GCSE History, but this CGP Topic Guide will help you answer exam questions with surgical precision.

It's packed with crystal-clear revision notes explaining the whole topic, plus plenty of useful activities, sample answers, exam tips and exam-style questions. You'll never get sick of it!

How to access your free Online Edition

This book includes a free Online Edition to read on your PC, Mac or tablet.
To access it, just go to **cgpbooks.co.uk/extras** and enter this code...

4232 5344 9861 4515

By the way, this code only works for one person. If somebody else has used this book before you, they might have already claimed the Online Edition.

CGP — still the best! ☺

Our sole aim here at CGP is to produce the highest quality books — carefully written, immaculately presented and dangerously close to being funny.

Then we work our socks off to get them out to you — at the cheapest possible prices.

Published by CGP

Editors:
Andy Cashmore, Robbie Driscoll, Catherine Heygate, Holly Robinson

With thanks to Sophie Herring for the proofreading.
With thanks to Emily Smith for the copyright research.

Acknowledgements:
With thanks to Getty Images for permission to use the image on the cover: © Science & Society Picture Library/ SSPL/ Getty Images.
With thanks to TopFoto for permission to use the image on page 5.
With thanks to Mary Evans Picture Library for permission to use the images on pages 6, 12, 16, 22, 24, 32, 42, 45, 50 and 52.

Extract on page 11 from 'Greco-Arab and Islamic Herbal Medicine: Traditional System, Ethics, Safety, Efficacy, and Regulatory Issues' by Bashar Saad and Omar Said. Copyright 2011 by John Wiley & Sons, Inc. All rights reserved.

Image on page 31: Crimean War: Florence Nightingale at Scutari Hospital. Coloured lithograph by E. Walker, 1856, after W. Simpson. Credit: Wellcome Collection https://wellcomecollection.org/works/ssfhw5uq This image is licensed under the CC BY 4.0 https://creativecommons.org/licenses/by/4.0/legalcode

Image on page 35: A monster being fed baskets of infants and excreting them with horns; symbolising vaccination and its effects. Etching by C. Williams, 1802(?). Credit: Wellcome Collection https://wellcomecollection.org/works/ssfhw5uq This image is licensed under the CC BY 4.0 https://creativecommons.org/licenses/by/4.0/legalcode

With thanks to Alamy for permission to use the images on pages 43 and 48.

Extract on page 55: Copyright Guardian News & Media Ltd 2019.

Image on page 59: 'The dawn of hope'. National insurance against sickness and disablement. Support the Liberal government in their policy of social reform'. / British Library, London, UK / © British Library Board. All Rights Reserved / Bridgeman Images.

Image on page 66 © Solo Syndication/ Associated Newspapers Ltd.

ISBN: 978 1 78908 284 5
Printed by Elanders Ltd, Newcastle upon Tyne.

Based on the classic CGP style created by Richard Parsons.

Contents

Exam Skills

Medicine Stands Still

The Beginnings of Change

A Revolution in Medicine

Modern Medicine

Exam Hints and Tips

GCSE AQA History is made up of two papers. The papers test different skills and each one covers different topics. This page gives you more information about each exam so you'll know what to expect.

You will take Two Papers altogether

Paper 1 covers the Period Study and the Wider World Depth Study

> It's really important that you make sure you know which topics you're studying for each paper.

Paper 1 is 2 hours long. It's worth 84 marks — 50% of your GCSE.
This paper will be divided into two sections:
- Section A: Period Study.
- Section B: Wider World Depth Study.

Paper 2 covers the Thematic Study and the British Depth Study

Paper 2 is 2 hours long. It's worth 84 marks — 50% of your GCSE.
This paper will be divided into two sections:
- Section A: Thematic Study. ◄
- Section B: British Depth Study. This also includes
  a question on the Historic Environment.

> This book covers the Thematic Study Britain: Health and the people: c1000 to the present day.

Thematic Studies are about Developments over a Long Period

1) The thematic studies cover a long period of history (around 1000 years). They focus on understanding how a certain topic has developed throughout different eras of British history.

2) You'll need to have a detailed knowledge of your topic — this means knowing the main developments and important events that took place. It also means understanding how important factors (e.g. individuals, the government, the Church and warfare) helped to shape events and developments.

3) You should know the significance of the main events and individuals really well. You also need to know the similarities and differences between developments in different periods, as well as the causes and consequences of the major changes throughout the period of the Thematic Study.

Thematic Studies include questions about Sources

1) Sources are pieces of evidence about the topic you're studying — such as a newspaper cartoon criticising Edward Jenner or an extract from a speech about the NHS by Aneurin Bevan.

2) Sources may also be someone's reflections on an issue or event they experienced, written or recorded after it took place. For example, a source could be an interview with someone who worked in a hospital during the Second World War, carried out after the war had ended.

3) Historians use sources to find out about and make sense of the past. They have to choose sources carefully to make sure they're useful for the specific question they are trying to answer.

4) Once they find a useful source, they use it to arrive at conclusions about the topic they're studying — this is called making inferences.

5) For the Thematic Study, you'll be asked to evaluate the usefulness of a source (see p.5).

Exam Hints and Tips

Remember these Tips for Approaching the Questions

Stay focused on the question

- Read the questions <u>carefully</u>. Underline the <u>key words</u> in each question so you know exactly what you need to do.
- Make sure that you <u>directly answer the question</u>. Don't just chuck in everything you know about medicine.
- You've got to be <u>relevant</u> and <u>accurate</u> — make sure you include <u>precise details</u> in your answers.
- It might help to try to write the <u>first sentence</u> of every <u>paragraph</u> in a way that <u>addresses</u> the question, e.g. "Another way modern surgery is similar to surgery in the Middle Ages is..."

> For example, you should include the <u>dates</u> of important events in the history of medicine and the <u>names</u> of the people who were involved.

Plan your essay answers

- You <u>don't</u> need to plan answers to the <u>shorter questions</u> in the exam.
- For the <u>long essay question</u>, it's very important to make a <u>quick plan</u> before you start writing. This will help to make your answer <u>well organised</u> and <u>structured</u>, with each point <u>leading clearly</u> to your <u>conclusion</u>.
- Look at the <u>key words</u> in the question. Scribble a <u>quick plan</u> of your <u>main points</u> — <u>cross through this neatly</u> at the end, so it's obvious it shouldn't be marked.

Organise your Time in the exam

1) Always double check that you know <u>how much time</u> you have for each paper.
2) <u>Learn the rule</u> — the <u>more marks</u> a question is worth, the <u>longer</u> your answer should be. The number of marks available for each question is clearly shown in the exam paper.
3) Try not to spend too much time on one question — you need to <u>leave enough time</u> so you can answer <u>all</u> of the questions.
4) Try to leave a few minutes at the <u>end</u> of the exam to go back and <u>read over</u> your answers.

Always use a Clear Writing Style

1) Try to use <u>clear handwriting</u> — and pay attention to <u>spelling</u>, <u>grammar</u> and <u>punctuation</u>.
2) If you make a mistake, miss out a word or need to add extra information to a point, make your changes <u>neatly</u>. Check that the examiner will still be able to <u>easily read</u> and <u>understand</u> your answer.
3) Remember to start a <u>new paragraph</u> for each new point you want to discuss.
4) A brief <u>introduction</u> and <u>conclusion</u> will help to give <u>structure</u> to your essay answers and make sure you stay <u>focused</u> on the <u>question</u>.

 ### *Use this page to make exam stress a thing of the past...*

Your spelling, grammar and punctuation are particularly important for the essay question at the end of the Thematic Study paper — there are four marks available for getting them right.

Skills for the Thematic Study

These two pages will give you some advice on how to approach the Thematic Study, as well as how to find your way around this book. Activity types are colour-coded to help you find what you need.

The Thematic Study tests Three different Skills

1) Throughout the Thematic Study, you'll be expected to show your knowledge and understanding of the topic, as well as your ability to apply historical concepts, such as cause and consequence.

2) For questions which ask you to analyse sources, you'll also need to use more specific skills.

3) The activities in this book will help you to practise all the different skills you'll need for the exam.

Knowledge and Understanding

1) You'll need to use your own knowledge and understanding of the topic to back up all your answers in the exam.

2) It's important that you use accurate and relevant information to support your ideas.

> The Knowledge and Understanding activities in this book will help you to revise key features and events from different periods — what was happening, when it was happening, who was involved and all the other important details.

Thinking Historically

1) As well as knowing what happened when, you'll also need to use historical concepts to analyse key events and developments. These concepts include significance, similarity and difference, cause, consequence and change.

> Explain why Germ Theory was important for the development of medicine.   [8 marks]

2) Question 2 in the exam will ask you to explain the importance of an individual, group, event or development in the history of medicine. Think about how they changed medicine in the short term and whether they caused any long-term changes.

3) Question 3 is all about similarities and/or differences between two events, developments, individuals or groups. For this question, make sure you cover a range of comparison points and explain why they make the two topics similar or different.

> Explain the similarities between public health in the 19th century and public health after the Second World War.   [8 marks]

4) Question 4 focuses on the role of factors like individuals, the government and warfare in the development of medicine. Decide your opinion before you start writing and state it clearly at the beginning and end of your answer. Don't forget to discuss a range of factors in your argument and use examples from across the whole period of the Thematic Study.

> Has war been the most important factor in the development of surgery since c.1000? Explain your answer.   [16 marks]

5) There are 4 marks available for spelling, punctuation, grammar and the use of specialist terminology for Question 4, so it's worth 20 marks in total.

> The Thinking Historically activities in this book will help you to practise using historical concepts to analyse different parts of the topic.

Skills for the Thematic Study

Source Analysis

1) Question 1 in the exam will be a source-based question. It will ask you to <u>explain</u> how <u>useful</u> a source would be for studying a particular aspect of medicine.

> Look at Source A. How useful would it be for studying attitudes towards the NHS? Use Source A and your own knowledge to explain your answer. [8 marks]

2) When you're answering this question, it's important that you write about the <u>provenance</u> of the source. This means discussing features like:
   - The <u>date</u> — when the source was produced
   - The <u>author</u> — who produced it
   - The <u>purpose</u> — why it might have been produced

3) In your answer, you need to explain how these factors affect the <u>usefulness</u> of the source for studying the topic given in the question.

4) You also need to write about the <u>content</u> of the source. It's important that you don't just <u>describe</u> what you can see or read in the source. You need to use your <u>own knowledge</u> to <u>analyse</u> how the content of the source affects its <u>usefulness</u>.

For example, the source on the right is a cartoon that was published in Punch magazine on 22nd December 1948.

The cartoon was published just a few months after the NHS was founded, so it is useful for studying attitudes towards the organisation immediately after its creation by Minister for Health Aneurin Bevan and the Labour government. In the cartoon, the doctor looks unhappy about his role as 'The Universal Provider', giving out gifts to a large crowd in his surgery. This is useful, because it suggests that even after its foundation the NHS faced ongoing opposition from some doctors. Before the NHS was created, many doctors opposed the new organisation, either because they were reluctant to be controlled by the government, or because they feared they would lose out financially. The government eventually managed to persuade doctors to accept the NHS by offering them a payment for each patient and allowing them to continue treating fee-paying patients. However, this source suggests that these measures did not fully convince all doctors, and that a few months after the NHS was founded some still had concerns about it.

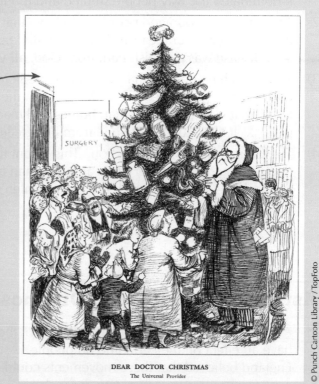

DEAR DOCTOR CHRISTMAS
The Universal Provider

© Punch Cartoon Library / TopFoto

5) You might be given a <u>written</u> source or a <u>visual</u> source in the exam — you should handle them both in the <u>same way</u>.

> The <u>Source Analysis</u> activities in this book will help you to practise <u>understanding</u> sources, <u>evaluating</u> what they are saying and analysing their <u>usefulness</u>.

Tomato sauce is useful for barbecue studies...

The Thematic Study might seem a bit scary because it covers such a long period of time, but don't worry — in this book the topic is broken down into different time periods to help you.

Disease and the Supernatural

In medieval England (and for the purposes of this section we're talking roughly 1000 to 1500), treatment of disease was a bit... medieval. The key problem was a lack of understanding of the causes of disease.

Disease was thought to have Supernatural Causes

1) Many people believed that disease was a punishment from God for people's sins. They thought that disease existed to show them the error of their ways and to make them become better people. Therefore, they thought that the way to cure disease was through prayer and repentance.

2) Disease was also thought to be caused by evil supernatural beings, like demons or witches. Witches were believed to be behind outbreaks of disease — many people were tried as witches and executed.

3) People believed that some diseases could be caused by evil spirits living inside someone. Members of the Church performed exorcisms, using chants to remove the spirit from the person's body.

The Church had a big Influence on medieval medicine

1) The Roman Catholic Church was an extremely powerful organisation in medieval Europe. It dominated the way people studied and thought about a range of topics, including medicine.

2) The Church encouraged people to believe that disease was a punishment from God, rather than having a natural cause. This prevented people from trying to find cures for disease — if disease was a punishment from God, all you could do was pray and repent.

3) The Church made sure that scholars of medicine learned the works of Galen (see p.8) as his ideas fit the Christian belief that God created human bodies and made them to be perfect. It also stopped anyone from disagreeing with Galen.

4) The Church outlawed dissection. This meant that medieval doctors couldn't discover ideas about human anatomy for themselves — they instead had to learn Galen's incorrect ideas.

Comment and Analysis

The Church's influence over medieval medicine meant that there was very little change in ideas about the cause of disease until the Renaissance — the Church and its messages were so influential that people were unable to question them.

Astrology was used to Diagnose disease

1) Astrology is the idea that the movements of the planets and stars have an effect on the Earth and on people. Astrologers in medieval England believed that these movements could cause disease.

2) Astrology was a new way of diagnosing disease. It was developed in Arabic medicine and brought to Europe between 1100 and 1300.

3) Medieval doctors owned a type of calendar (called an almanac) which included information about where particular planets and stars were at any given time. The doctor then used this information to predict how patients' health could be affected.

4) Different star signs were thought to affect different parts of the body.

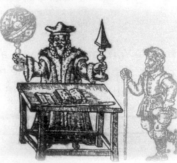

A woodcut from 1490 showing two astrologers looking at the positions of the Sun and Moon.

© Photo Researchers / Mary Evans Picture Library

Disease and the Supernatural

Medieval people often believed that disease had supernatural causes, such as God, witches or evil spirits. Try these activities to make sure you know the different theories about the causes of disease.

Knowledge and Understanding

1) Copy and complete the table below, explaining how medieval people dealt with the following 'causes' of disease.

Cause	How people dealt with it
a) Punishment from God	
b) Witches	
c) Evil spirits	

2) How was astrology used by doctors to diagnose disease?

Thinking Historically

1) Copy and complete the mind map below, adding points about the different ways that the Church influenced medieval medicine.

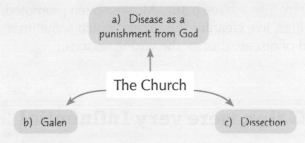

a) Disease as a punishment from God

The Church

b) Galen

c) Dissection

2) Which of the three aspects mentioned above do you think was most responsible for preventing medical developments during the medieval period? Explain your answer.

3) Do you think astrology was significant in changing medieval attitudes to the causes of disease? Explain your answer.

EXAM TIP

The medieval period — a dark age for medicine...

It's important to understand medieval people's beliefs about the causes of disease. In the exam, you might get a question asking how these beliefs compare to later periods.

Medicine Stands Still

Natural Explanations

Some treatments in medieval Britain were based <u>less</u> on <u>religious faith</u> and <u>more</u> on <u>natural theories</u> and observation of the physical world. But a reason-based theory can still be <u>wrong</u>.

Medicine was dominated by the Four Humours Theory

After the fall of the <u>Roman Empire</u>, much Ancient <u>Greek</u> and <u>Roman</u> medical knowledge was <u>lost</u> in the West. The <u>Theory of the Four Humours</u> was eventually brought back to western Europe via the <u>Islamic world</u> (see p.10). Many medieval doctors based their <u>diagnosis</u> and <u>treatment</u> on this theory.

1) The Theory of the <u>Four Humours</u> was created by the Ancient Greek doctor <u>Hippocrates</u> (c.460-c.377 BC). Hippocrates believed that the body was made up of <u>four fluids</u> (or <u>humours</u>) — <u>blood</u>, <u>phlegm</u>, <u>yellow bile</u> and <u>black bile</u>. These were linked to the <u>four seasons</u> and the <u>four elements</u>. They needed to be in <u>balance</u> for good health.

> E.g. in winter we get colds. So Hippocrates thought that in winter the body created an excess of <u>phlegm</u>. Sadly, Hippocrates failed to see that a bunged up nose, fevers, etc. are <u>symptoms</u> of the disease — he thought they were the <u>cause</u>.

> E.g. someone with a <u>cold</u> (too much cold, wet <u>phlegm</u>) could be given chicken, pepper or wine (all considered <u>hot</u> and <u>dry</u>) to correct the <u>imbalance</u>.

2) The Theory of the Four Humours was developed further by another Greek doctor, <u>Galen</u>, who was born in AD 129 and worked for much of his career in <u>Rome</u>.

3) Galen believed that diseases could be treated using <u>opposites</u>. He thought that different foods, drinks, herbs and spices had a <u>humour</u>, which could <u>balance</u> the excessive humour that was causing the disease.

The Miasma Theory blamed Bad Air for causing disease

1) The <u>miasma</u> theory is the idea that <u>bad air</u> (or miasma) causes disease when someone breathes it in. This bad air may come from human <u>waste</u> or <u>dead bodies</u> — anything that creates a <u>bad smell</u>.

2) The miasma theory originated in Ancient <u>Greece</u> and <u>Rome</u>, and was incorporated by <u>Galen</u> into the Theory of the Four Humours. The idea became extremely popular in medieval Britain.

3) The miasma theory was so influential that it lasted until the <u>1860s</u>, when it was replaced by the <u>Germ Theory</u> (see p.36). Miasma often prompted people to do <u>hygienic</u> things, like cleaning the streets, which sometimes helped to stop the spread of disease (but for the wrong reasons).

> **Comment and Analysis**
>
> The Four Humours and miasma were both <u>incorrect</u> theories. But they assumed disease had a <u>natural</u> cause, rather than a supernatural one. This was important, as it suggested that people weren't <u>powerless</u> against disease — they could <u>investigate</u> and <u>take action</u> against it.

Hippocrates and Galen were very Influential

The work of Hippocrates and <u>Galen</u> was extremely influential in medical diagnosis and treatment.

1) Hippocrates and Galen wrote down their beliefs about medicine. These were <u>translated</u> into Latin books, which were considered important texts by the <u>Roman Catholic Church</u>. Like the Bible, Hippocrates' and Galen's ideas were considered the <u>absolute truth</u>.

2) Many of their ideas were taught for <u>centuries</u> after their deaths, including the <u>incorrect</u> ones. For example, Galen only ever dissected <u>animals</u> — animal and human bodies are very different, so some of his ideas about <u>anatomy</u> were <u>wrong</u>. Medieval doctors were <u>not allowed</u> to perform their own dissections, so they continued to learn Galen's incorrect ideas.

3) Some of Hippocrates' and Galen's ideas were so influential that they continue to be used <u>today</u>. The <u>Hippocratic Oath</u> is the <u>promise</u> made by doctors to obey rules of behaviour in their professional lives — a version of it is still in use today. Hippocrates and Galen also believed that doctors should <u>observe</u> their patients as they treat them.

Natural Explanations

These activities will help you understand natural explanations for disease during the medieval period.

Knowledge and Understanding

1) Using your own words, explain each of the headings in the boxes below.

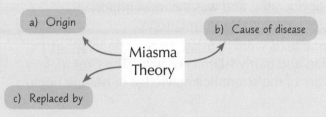

a) Hippocrates' Theory of the Four Humours

b) How Galen developed the theory

2) Explain why a medieval doctor might have told someone with a cold to drink some wine.

3) Copy and complete the mind map below to explain what the miasma theory is.

a) Origin

Miasma Theory

b) Cause of disease

c) Replaced by

4) Explain why the miasma theory sometimes helped prevent disease, even though it was incorrect.

Thinking Historically

1) Copy and complete the diagram below, explaining how each of the points affected medieval medicine.

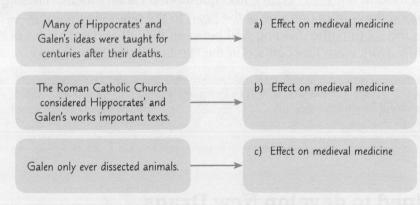

Many of Hippocrates' and Galen's ideas were taught for centuries after their deaths.

a) Effect on medieval medicine

The Roman Catholic Church considered Hippocrates' and Galen's works important texts.

b) Effect on medieval medicine

Galen only ever dissected animals.

c) Effect on medieval medicine

2) Do you think Hippocrates and Galen were the most important influences on medieval medicine in Britain? Explain your answer.

The four humours — they're totally hilarious...

In the exam, it's important to take a couple of minutes before the start of the longer question to plan your answer. This will make sure that you answer the question and don't veer off topic.

Islamic Medicine

In the medieval period, Islamic medicine was miles ahead of European medicine. Arabic ideas eventually made their way to Europe — including knowledge of the all-important Galen and Hippocrates.

Arab doctors kept Classical Knowledge alive

1) While a lot of medical knowledge was lost in the West after the fall of the Roman Empire, medical ideas like the Four Humours and treatment by opposites (see p.8) were kept alive by Islamic scholars.

2) In the 9th century, Hunain ibn Ishaq (also known by his Latin name Johannitius) travelled from Baghdad to Byzantium to collect Greek medical texts. He translated these into Arabic.

3) This classical knowledge was eventually brought to Europe by Avicenna (or Ibn Sina), a Persian who lived from around AD 980-1037. Avicenna wrote the 'Canon of Medicine', which brought together the ideas of Galen and Hippocrates, and was the most important way that classical ideas got back into Western Europe.

4) This work and other Islamic texts were translated into Latin in Spain (which was partly Christian and partly Islamic) or Italy. The Crusades also made Europeans aware of the scientific knowledge of Islamic doctors.

> **Comment and Analysis**
>
> Islamic medicine was generally more rational and evidence-based than European medicine, partly due to their knowledge of classical (Ancient Greek and Roman) medical texts.

> The Crusades were a series of wars fought by Christian Europeans against Muslims. They were an ultimately unsuccessful attempt to retake Jerusalem and the surrounding areas associated with the early history of Christianity.

Islamic doctors made several New Discoveries

1) Albucasis (or Abu al-Qasim, born c.AD 936) wrote a well thought-out book describing amputations, the removal of bladder stones and dental surgery — as well as methods for handling fractures, dislocations and the stitching of wounds.

2) In the 12th century, Avenzoar (or Ibn Zuhr) described the parasite that causes scabies and began to question the reliability of Galen.

3) Ibn al-Nafis, who lived in the 13th century, also questioned Galen's ideas. He suggested (correctly) that blood flows from one side of the heart to the other via the lungs — and doesn't cross the septum (the dividing wall between the left and right sides of the heart). Ibn al-Nafis' work wasn't recognised in the West until the 20th century.

> **Comment and Analysis**
>
> In the Islamic world, as in Western Europe, religion strongly influenced the development of medicine. For example, Islam, like Christianity, prohibited dissection.

> The autobiography of Usama ibn Munqidh, a 12th century Muslim doctor, suggests the difference between Islamic and European medicine. Usama describes how he treated a knight with a sore on his leg by using a poultice, and a woman who was 'feeble-minded' by advising a new diet. Then a French doctor arrived and claimed Usama knew nothing. He cut off the knight's leg with an axe, and cut the woman's head with a razor and rubbed the skull with salt. Both patients died.

Alchemy helped to develop New Drugs

1) Alchemy was the attempt to turn base (ordinary) metals into gold and to discover the elixir of eternal life.

2) Alchemy traces its origins back to the Egyptians and it was preserved in the Islamic world.

3) Unlike modern chemistry, much superstition was included — an unsuccessful experiment was as likely to be blamed on the position of the stars or the spiritual purity of the alchemist as anything else.

4) Even so, Arabic alchemists invented useful techniques such as distillation and sublimation, and prepared drugs such as laudanum, benzoin and camphor.

Islamic Medicine

SKILLS PRACTICE

Check that you know how Islamic medicine and European medicine compared with these activities.

Knowledge and Understanding

1) Using the key words below, explain how Islamic doctors were important in keeping classical knowledge alive in the medieval period.

Roman Empire   Johannitius   Avicenna   'Canon of Medicine'

2) Describe the contribution made to medieval medicine by the following people:

a) Albucasis   b) Avenzoar   c) Ibn al-Nafis

3) Why was alchemy important in the development of medicine?

Thinking Historically

1) Copy and complete the table below, giving the similarities and differences between Islamic medicine and European medicine in the medieval period.

Use information from pages 6-10 to help you.

Similarities	Differences

Source Analysis

The source below is from a book by Rhazes, an Islamic scientist who was alive in the 9th century.

> It grieves me to oppose and criticise the man, Galen, from whose sea of knowledge I have drawn much. <u>Indeed, he is the Master and I am the disciple</u>. Although this reverence* and appreciation will and <u>should not prevent me from doubting, as I did, what is erroneous** in his theories</u>. I imagine and feel deeply in my heart that Galen has chosen me to undertake this task, and if he were alive, he would have congratulated me on what I am doing.

a)

b)

*respect   **incorrect

1) Explain what each highlighted phrase suggests about Rhazes' attitude towards Galen.

2) Imagine you are using this source for an investigation into medieval attitudes towards Galen. Explain how the features of the source below affect its usefulness for your investigation.

a) Author   b) Content

EXAM TIP

I'm an alchemist — I turn revision guides into gold...

Before attempting the source question in the exam, look at the source carefully to make sure you understand the point it's making. Highlighting key features or quotes can help you do this.

Treating Disease

As the Middle Ages went on, medical treatments continued to be based on ideas we'd nowadays consider very <u>unscientific</u>. <u>Treatments</u> were <u>ambitious</u> though, and <u>theories</u> quite <u>sophisticated</u> in their <u>own ways</u>.

Prayer and Repentance were major treatments

1) Disease was believed to be a punishment from God, so sick people were encouraged to <u>pray</u>. The sick often prayed to <u>saints</u>, in the hope they would intervene and stop the illness. Medieval people also believed that <u>pilgrimages</u> to <u>holy shrines</u> (e.g. sites containing the remains of saints) could cure <u>illnesses</u>.

2) Others took their <u>repentance</u> one step further. <u>Flagellants</u> were people who whipped themselves in public in order to show God that they were sorry for their past actions. They were particularly common during <u>epidemics</u>, such as the Black Death (see p.18).

3) Many <u>doctors</u> had <u>superstitious beliefs</u> — e.g. some used <u>astrology</u> to diagnose and treat illness (see p.6), or believed that saying <u>certain words</u> while giving a treatment could make that treatment more effective.

Bloodletting and Purging aimed to make the Humours balanced

1) <u>Bloodletting</u> and <u>purging</u> were popular treatments because they fitted in with the <u>Four Humours Theory</u>.

2) If someone apparently had too much blood inside them, the doctor would take blood out of their body through <u>bloodletting</u> — they might make a small <u>cut</u> to remove the blood or use blood-sucking <u>leeches</u>.

3) Some people were accidentally <u>killed</u> because too much blood was taken.

4) <u>Purging</u> is the act of getting rid of other fluids from the body by <u>excreting</u> — doctors gave their patients <u>laxatives</u> to help the purging process.

Comment and Analysis

<u>Bloodletting</u> caused more deaths than it prevented, but it remained a popular treatment. This shows the strength of medieval people's <u>beliefs</u> in the face of <u>observational evidence</u>.

Purifying the Air was thought to Prevent Disease

1) The <u>miasma</u> theory (see p.8) led people to believe in the power of <u>purifying</u> or <u>cleaning</u> the air to prevent sickness and improve health.

2) Physicians carried <u>posies</u> or <u>oranges</u> around with them when visiting patients to protect themselves from catching a disease.

3) During the <u>Black Death</u> (see p.18), <u>juniper</u>, <u>myrrh</u> and <u>incense</u> were burned so the <u>smoke</u> or <u>scent</u> would <u>fill the room</u> and stop bad air from bringing disease <u>inside</u>.

Purifying the air was also seen as important for helping with <u>other health conditions</u>. In the case of <u>fainting</u>, people <u>burned feathers</u> and made the patient <u>breathe in their smoke</u>.

Remedies were Early Natural Medicines

1) Remedies bought from an <u>apothecary</u>, local <u>wise woman</u> or made at <u>home</u> were all popular in medieval Britain and contained <u>herbs</u>, <u>spices</u>, <u>animal parts</u> and <u>minerals</u>.

2) These remedies were either <u>passed down</u> or <u>written</u> in books explaining how to mix them together. Some of these books were called 'Herbals'.

3) Other remedies were based on <u>superstition</u>, like <u>lucky charms</u> containing 'powdered unicorn's horn'.

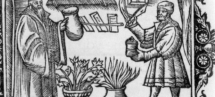

© Mary Evans Picture Library

This medieval print shows a doctor and an apothecary. The plants in the middle show the importance of herbal remedies.

Treating Disease

Now that you know all about how diseases were treated in the Middle Ages, have a go at these activities.

Knowledge and Understanding

1) Copy and complete the mind map below, adding points about the different ways that people in the medieval period treated disease.

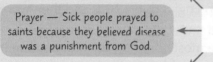

Prayer — Sick people prayed to saints because they believed disease was a punishment from God.

Treatment of disease

2) Bloodletting caused more deaths than it prevented. Why do you think medieval doctors continued to use this treatment even though it was unsafe?

Thinking Historically

1) Explain how belief in the Theory of the Four Humours and the miasma theory affected medical treatments in the medieval period.

2) Copy and complete the table below by listing evidence for and against each statement about medical treatments in the medieval period.

Statement	Evidence for	Evidence against
a) 'Religion was the biggest influence on medical treatments in the medieval period.'		
b) 'Medieval people mostly made medical treatments from things they found in the world around them.'		
c) 'Medical treatments in the medieval period usually caused more harm than good.'		

3) Explain whether, overall, you agree or disagree with each statement in the table above.

Medieval medical treatment was varied and diverse...

You might get a question in the exam on the similarities or differences between medical treatments in the medieval period and a later period — so make sure you know them well.

Treating Disease

If you were ill in the Middle Ages, you couldn't just go to your local GP. But as there were various kinds of medical healers, there could still be an element of 'patient choice'...

People used lots of Different Healers

1) Physicians were male doctors who had trained at university for at least seven years. They read ancient texts as well as writings from the Islamic world (see p.10) but their training involved little practical experience. They used handbooks (vademecums) and clinical observation to check patients' conditions. But there were fewer than 100 physicians in England in 1300, and they were very expensive.

2) Most people saw an apothecary, who prepared and sold remedies (see p.12), and gave advice on how best to use them. Apothecaries were the most common form of treatment in Britain as they were the most accessible for those who could not afford a physician.

3) Apothecaries were trained through apprenticeships. Most apothecaries were men, but there were also many so-called 'wise women', who sold herbal remedies.

There were Few Public Hospitals

1) Most public hospitals were set up and run by the Church. There were relatively few such hospitals, but they were very popular and highly regarded.

2) The main purpose of hospitals was not to treat disease, but to care for the sick and elderly. The hospital provided its patients with food, water and a warm place to stay. Most hospitals were also more hygienic than elsewhere, because they had developed water and sewerage systems.

3) Some monasteries also cared for the sick, the elderly or the poor (see p.16).

4) Most sick people were treated at home by members of their family.

> Famous hospitals like St. Bartholomew's and St. Thomas' in London started life as church establishments. The monastery at Canterbury Cathedral already had a complex water and sanitation system by 1250.

Surgery — work for Barbers, not doctors

1) Medieval surgery was very dangerous — there was no way to prevent blood loss, infection or pain. It was therefore only attempted rarely and for very minor procedures, e.g. treating hernias or cataracts.

2) There were a few university-trained, highly paid surgeons, but surgery as a whole was not a respected profession in medieval times — most operations were carried out by barber-surgeons (who also cut hair).

Some Progress was made in Surgery

1) Hugh of Lucca and his son Theodoric worked as surgeons in Italy in the early 13th century. They recognised the importance of practical experience and observation, and questioned some of Galen's ideas — their thoughts appear in Theodoric's textbooks.

2) They began dressing wounds with bandages soaked in wine, because they noticed that the wine helped to keep wounds clean and prevent infection. They made this discovery by chance.

Comment and Analysis

Hugh and Theodoric's approach was unusual in the Middle Ages. It wasn't until the Renaissance that people started to question widely-held beliefs about the causes of disease, and to carry out experiments to find more effective methods of treatment and prevention.

3) They also realised that pus was not a healthy sign, unlike other doctors at the time who might try to cause wounds to pus because they believed it would release toxins from the body.

4) Some surgeons tried to find ways to reduce pain during operations. For example, John of Arderne created a recipe for an anaesthetic in 1376 which included hemlock, opium and henbane (a relative of deadly nightshade). In carefully controlled doses this may have worked — but was very likely to kill.

Treating Disease

There were different kinds of healers in medieval times, but they all had their limitations. The activities on this page will help test your knowledge of each type.

Knowledge and Understanding

1) Copy and complete the table below by adding as much detail as possible about each type of healer.

Physician	Apothecary	Barber-Surgeon

2) For each person listed below, write down the type of healer or medical institution they might have visited to get treatment. Explain your answers.

   a) A poor person with a hernia

   b) A rich person with a headache

   c) A sick, elderly person with no family to support them

   d) A poor person with a cough

3) Describe three developments in wound treatment and surgery in the period c.1200-c.1400.

4) Explain how Hugh and Theodoric of Lucca's work was ahead of its time.

Thinking Historically

1) Write down a piece of evidence for and against each statement in the boxes below.

   a) 'Access to medical treatments was similar for both rich and poor people in the medieval period.'

   b) 'Hospitals in the medieval period had a big impact on helping people to get better.'

   c) 'The main reason why surgery was dangerous in the medieval period was because few operations were carried out by university-trained surgeons.'

2) Explain how each of the following type of healer affected progress in treating diseases during the medieval period:

   a) Physicians

   b) Apothecaries

   Use the information on page 12 to help you with part b) of question 2.

EXAM TIP

Anyone can be a barber-surgeon — it's not brain surgery...

Some of your marks in the exam are for using specialist terminology. Make sure you use specific terms in your exam, e.g. say 'vademecum' (if you can spell it) instead of 'handbook'.

Health in Towns and Monasteries

In the medieval period, how healthy people were had a lot do with the area where they lived.

Living Conditions in Towns were pretty Poor

1) Houses in towns were usually made of wood and were crammed together — overcrowding and fires were common problems.

2) A lot of towns didn't have clean water supplies or sewerage systems — waste was chucked into the street or into rivers to be washed away. Sewage from latrines (pits with wooden seats) leaked into the ground and got into wells.

> 'When passing along the water of Thames, we have beheld dung and lay stools and other filth accumulated in diverse places within the city, and have also perceived the fumes and other abominable stenches arising therefrom...' King Edward III commenting on the state of the Thames in London in 1357.

3) Businesses and homes weren't separated — butchers, tanners and dyers threw toxic waste into rivers and residential streets. People had to get their drinking water from rivers and wells that were contaminated.

4) In the 13th century, a water channel called the Great Conduit was built to bring clean water into London, as the Thames was getting too toxic.

5) In 1388, the government ordered town authorities to keep the streets free of waste. Towns introduced public health measures to tackle waste, sewage and pollution and to create a clean water supply.

York and London both banned people from dumping waste in the street. These cities also built latrines over rivers so that sewage could be carried away.

London eventually banned any waste from being thrown into the Thames — carters were hired to collect waste and take it out of the city.

Many towns, like York, ordered toxic businesses like butchers, tanners, fishmongers and dyers to move outside the city walls.

Comment and Analysis

People broke these rules and officials struggled to enforce them. People knew that dirty water and bad health were linked, but they didn't really understand the risks. Town authorities didn't have enough money or knowledge to properly fix these public health issues.

Monasteries were Healthier than Towns

Monasteries had cleaner water than towns and had good systems for getting rid of waste and sewage. Monks also had access to books on healing and they knew how to grow herbs and make herbal remedies.

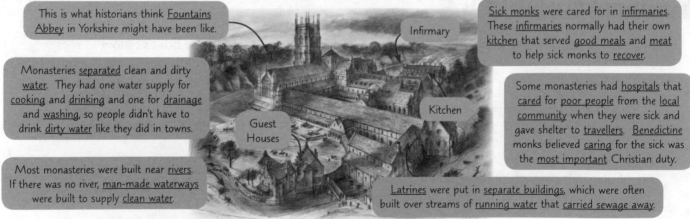

This is what historians think Fountains Abbey in Yorkshire might have been like.

Monasteries separated clean and dirty water. They had one water supply for cooking and drinking and one for drainage and washing, so people didn't have to drink dirty water like they did in towns.

Most monasteries were built near rivers. If there was no river, man-made waterways were built to supply clean water.

Infirmary

Sick monks were cared for in infirmaries. These infirmaries normally had their own kitchen that served good meals and meat to help sick monks to recover.

Some monasteries had hospitals that cared for poor people from the local community when they were sick and gave shelter to travellers. Benedictine monks believed caring for the sick was the most important Christian duty.

Kitchen

Guest Houses

Latrines were put in separate buildings, which were often built over streams of running water that carried sewage away.

© Historic England / Mary Evans

It was easier to create healthy living conditions in monasteries than it was in towns.

1) Monasteries were wealthy, so they could afford to build infrastructure like latrine buildings and waterways to keep their water clean. Towns had to rely on wealthy individuals to fund these kinds of projects.

2) Monastery populations were small and had one leader (the abbot) — he had the power to enforce rules about cleanliness and waste disposal. Getting hundreds of townspeople to adopt cleaner habits was trickier — towns didn't have one person in charge who could easily enforce public health measures.

Health in Towns and Monasteries

There were many reasons why the living conditions in towns and monasteries were different. The activities on this page will make sure you know the differences between towns and monasteries in the Middle Ages.

Knowledge and Understanding

1) Explain how each of the following were treated differently by towns and monasteries.
   a) Clean water
   b) Sewage disposal

2) Copy and complete the mind map below, explaining how each factor affected living conditions in towns and monasteries.

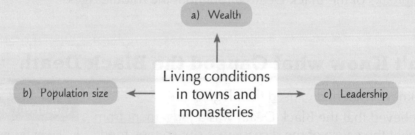

a) Wealth

Living conditions in towns and monasteries

b) Population size

c) Leadership

3) How did the government try to improve public health in towns in the Middle Ages?

Source Analysis

The source below is from a law about waste disposal that was written and passed by members of Parliament in 1388. This law applied to cities and towns in England, including London.

> ... so much dung and filth of the garbage and entrails... [are] cast and put into ditches, rivers, and other waters... that the air there is grown greatly corrupt and infected, and many maladies* and other intolerable diseases do daily happen... all they who do cast and lay all such annoyances, dung, garbages, entrails, and other ordure**, in ditches, rivers, waters, and other places aforesaid***, shall... forfeit to our Lord the King the sum of 20 pounds.

*illnesses   **dung   ***mentioned before

1) Imagine you are using this source for an investigation into public health in the Middle Ages. Explain how the features of the source below affect its usefulness for your investigation.

a) Content   b) Date   c) Purpose

The Black Death in Britain

The Black Death first struck in the 14th century. People tried to limit its spread, but couldn't stop the disease.

The Black Death was a devastating Epidemic

1) The Black Death was a series of plagues that swept Europe in the 14th century. It was really two illnesses:

- Bubonic plague, spread by the bites of fleas from rats carried on ships. This caused headaches and a high temperature, followed by pus-filled swellings on the skin.
- Pneumonic plague was airborne — it was spread by coughs and sneezes. It attacked the lungs, making it painful to breathe and causing victims to cough up blood.

2) The disease first arrived in Britain in 1348. Some historians think at least a third of the British population died as a result of the Black Death in 1348-50. There were further outbreaks of the Black Death throughout the Middle Ages.

People Didn't Know what Caused the Black Death

No-one at the time knew what had caused the plague.

1) Some people believed that the Black Death was a judgement from God. They thought the cause of the disease was sin, so they tried to prevent the spread of the disease through prayer and fasting.

2) Some blamed humour imbalances, so tried to get rid of the Black Death through bloodletting and purging. Those who thought that the disease was caused by miasma (see p.8) carried strong smelling herbs or lit fires to purify the air.

3) Some people also carried charms or used 'magic' potions containing arsenic.

Comment and Analysis

One of the main reasons why the Black Death killed so many was because people didn't know what caused the disease. Their ideas about the cause of disease were wrong, so their attempts at prevention and treatment were mostly ineffective.

Local Governments tried to Prevent the spread of the disease

1) Some people in Winchester thought that you could catch the plague from being close to the bodies of dead victims. When the town's cemetery became too full to take any more plague victims, the townspeople refused to let the bishop extend the cemetery in the town centre. Instead, they insisted that new cemeteries be built outside of the town, away from the houses.

2) The town of Gloucester tried to shut itself off from the outside world after hearing the Black Death had reached Bristol. This suggests that they thought the plague was spread by human contact. Their attempt at prevention was unsuccessful — many people in the town died of the Black Death.

3) In November 1348, the disease reached London. In January 1349, King Edward III closed Parliament.

The Black Death caused Social Change

1) After the Black Death, there were far fewer workers around. This meant that they could demand higher wages from their employers, and move around to find better work. The cost of land also decreased, allowing some peasants to buy land for the first time.

2) These changes threatened the power of the elites. The government created laws, such as the 1349 Ordinance of Labourers, to try and stop peasants moving around the country.

3) Some people think the Black Death helped cause the Peasants' Revolt in 1381, and, eventually, the collapse of the feudal system in Britain.

The Black Death in Britain

Try these activities about the Black Death, people's ideas about its causes and how they tried to stop it.

Knowledge and Understanding

1) Copy and complete the table below about the two types of plague that were part of the Black Death. For each one, describe how it was spread and its main symptoms.

Type of plague	How was it spread?	Symptoms
a) Bubonic Plague		
b) Pneumonic Plague		

2) When did the Black Death arrive in Britain and what effect did it have on the size of the population?

Thinking Historically

1) Copy and complete the mind map below by listing the different actions taken by the king, individuals, and local governments and communities in response to the Black Death. Include as much detail as you can.

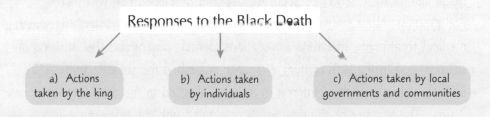

Responses to the Black Death

a) Actions taken by the king

b) Actions taken by individuals

c) Actions taken by local governments and communities

2) How do you think each of the following contributed to ineffective treatments for the Black Death? Explain your answers.

a) The influence of the Church
b) Lack of scientific knowledge
c) Superstitious beliefs

3) Why do you think medieval people were so powerless to stop the Black Death? Explain your answer.

4) Explain the consequences of the Black Death for each of the following groups of people:

a) workers
b) peasants
c) elites

Nobody really knew how to stop the Black Death...

EXAM TIP

Don't forget that the 14th century is referring to the 1300s. If you often get your centuries mixed up, try writing out the dates of an exam question in numbers above the words.

Medicine Stands Still

Worked Exam-Style Question

Have a look at this sample answer to give you an idea of how to approach question 2 in the exam.

Explain why Islamic medicine was important in the Middle Ages.   [8 marks]

The first sentence of each paragraph should address the question.

Islamic medicine was important in the Middle Ages because Islamic doctors were responsible for bringing Ancient Greek and Roman ideas about medicine back to Western Europe after the fall of the Roman Empire. In the 9th century, the Islamic scholar Johannitius collected Greek medical texts and translated them into Arabic. Avicenna used this classical knowledge to produce a text called 'the Canon of Medicine' which brought together the ideas of Galen and Hippocrates. Avicenna's work and other texts were then translated into Latin in Spain, which was partly Christian and partly Islamic, or in Italy. From here, the ideas of Hippocrates and Galen, such as the Theory of the Four Humours and the miasma theory, eventually reached Britain. This was hugely important because these theories influenced medicine in Europe for hundreds of years. People in Europe only began to question the Theory of the Four Humours during the Renaissance period, and the miasma theory was so influential that people continued to believe it until the 1860s when Pasteur developed the Germ Theory.

The answer looks at the importance of Islamic medicine in the long term.

Using specific facts and details shows a good understanding of the period.

Islamic medicine was important in the Middle Ages because Islamic doctors made significant discoveries about disease and developed new treatments. For example, Albucasis, who was born in c.936, wrote a book describing various medical treatments, including amputations, dental surgery and the stitching of wounds, and in the 12th century, Avenzoar described the parasite that causes scabies. Islamic doctors' interest in alchemy also led to the development of new drugs. The practice of alchemy, which originated with the Ancient Egyptians, was preserved in the Islamic world. Although alchemy relied heavily on superstition, Arabic alchemists still managed to invent useful medical techniques, such as distillation and sublimation, as well as preparing drugs like laudanum, benzoin and camphor. Therefore, alchemists and doctors in the Islamic world played an important role in improving the understanding of diseases and developing new medical methods and treatments.

The explanation links the point back to the question.

The answer covers different ways that Islamic medicine was important in the Middle Ages.

Islamic doctors such as Avenzoar and Ibn al-Nafis were also important because they began questioning the ideas of Galen. For example, in the 13th century, Ibn al-Nafis correctly suggested that blood flows from one side of the heart to the other via the lungs without crossing the septum. This differed from Galen, whose incorrect ideas about human anatomy had come from dissecting animals. However, the work of Islamic doctors had little impact on medicine in Europe in the Middle Ages. It was only when doctors such as Vesalius and Harvey began to carry out dissections in the Renaissance period that people in Western Europe started questioning Galen's ideas and identifying his mistakes.

Exam-Style Questions

Have a go at these exam-style questions to put everything you've learnt in this section into practice.

Source A

An account from 1349 about the behaviour of flagellants in London during the Black Death. The account was given by Sir Robert of Avesbury, an English historian.

Each [person] wore a cap marked with a red cross in front and behind. Each had in his right hand a scourge* with three tails. Each tail had a knot and through the middle of it there were sometimes sharp nails fixed. They marched naked in a file one behind the other and whipped themselves with these scourges on their naked and bleeding bodies... This went on from the first to the last until each of them had observed the ritual... Then each put on his customary garments and always wearing their caps and carrying their whips in their hands they retired to their lodgings. It is said that every night they performed the same penance.

*whip

Exam-Style Questions

1) Look at Source A. How useful would it be for studying responses to the Black Death? Use Source A and your own knowledge to explain your answer.   [8 marks]

2) Explain why natural explanations of disease were important in the Middle Ages.   [8 marks]

3) Explain the differences between public health in towns and monasteries in the Middle Ages.   [8 marks]

4) Has the Church been the most important factor in developments in the treatment of disease since the Middle Ages? Explain your answer.

For the 16-mark question in the exam, 4 extra marks will be available for spelling, punctuation, grammar and using specialist terminology.

Your answer should discuss the role of the Church and other factors. Make sure you include examples from across the period c.1000 to the present day.   [16 marks]

The Renaissance

The Renaissance was a time of <u>new ideas</u> and fresh <u>thinking</u>. People began to <u>challenge</u> old beliefs, and put forward <u>new theories</u> — such as <u>Vesalius'</u> ideas about <u>practical observation</u>.

The Renaissance was a time of Continuity and Change

1) In the Renaissance there was a <u>rediscovery</u> of knowledge from classical <u>Greek</u> and <u>Roman</u> times. Western doctors gained access to the original writings of <u>Hippocrates</u>, <u>Galen</u> and <u>Avicenna</u> (a Persian physician who lived between 980 and 1037 AD). These <u>hadn't been available</u> in the medieval period. They led to <u>greater interest</u> in the <u>Four Humours</u> Theory and <u>treatment by opposites</u> (see p.8).

2) But the Renaissance also saw the emergence of <u>science</u> as we know it from the <u>magic</u> and <u>mysticism</u> of medieval medicine. People thought about how the human body worked based on <u>direct observation</u> and <u>experimentation</u>.

3) This was partly because many of the new books that had been found said that <u>anatomy</u> and <u>dissections</u> were very important. This encouraged people to <u>examine</u> the body themselves, and to come to their <u>own conclusions</u> about the causes of disease.

4) People began to <u>question</u> Galen's thinking and that of other ancient doctors. However, his writings <u>continued to be studied</u>.

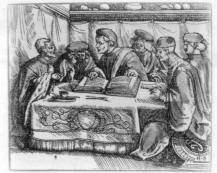

This woodcut shows physicians debating over a medicine book.

Protestant Christianity spread to Britain in the 16th century, during the <u>Reformation</u>. This reduced the influence of the <u>Catholic Church</u> in many areas of people's lives, including medicine. Although <u>religion</u> was still <u>important</u>, the Church no longer had so much control over medical teaching.

Vesalius wrote Anatomy books with Accurate Diagrams

1) <u>Vesalius</u> was born in <u>1514</u> and was a medical <u>professor</u> at Padua University, Italy. He believed that <u>successful surgery</u> would only be possible if doctors had a proper <u>understanding</u> of the <u>anatomy</u>.

2) Vesalius was able to perform <u>dissections</u> on <u>criminals</u> who had been <u>executed</u>. This let him study the human anatomy more closely.

3) He wrote books based on his observations using <u>accurate diagrams</u> to illustrate his work. The most important were 'Six Anatomical Pictures' (1538) and 'The Fabric of the Human Body' (1543).

> <u>Printing</u> was invented in the <u>1440s</u>, and the first <u>British printing press</u> was set up in the <u>1470s</u>. The invention of printing meant books could be <u>copied</u> more easily. This allowed new ideas to be shared and old ideas (e.g. Galen's theories) to be <u>discussed</u> and <u>questioned</u>.

4) His works were <u>printed</u> and <u>distributed</u> around Europe, including to <u>Britain</u>. This allowed <u>British doctors</u> to read about Vesalius' findings and <u>learn</u> from his <u>discoveries</u>.

5) Vesalius' work helped point out some of <u>Galen's mistakes</u>. For example, in the second edition of 'The Fabric', he showed that there were <u>no holes</u> in the septum of the heart.

6) His findings encouraged others to <u>question Galen</u>. Doctors also realised there was <u>more to discover</u> about the body because of Vesalius' <u>questioning</u> attitude.

7) Vesalius showed that <u>dissecting bodies</u> was important, to find out exactly how the human body was <u>structured</u>. Dissection was used <u>more and more</u> in medical training for this reason (see p.28).

Comment and Analysis

The work of Vesalius <u>didn't</u> have an immediate impact on the <u>diagnosis</u> or <u>treatment</u> of disease. However, by producing a realistic description of the human <u>anatomy</u> and encouraging <u>dissection</u>, Vesalius provided an essential <u>first step</u> to improving them.

The Renaissance

While the teachings of influential individuals such as Galen continued to be studied in the Renaissance, new ideas were being introduced by people like Vesalius. Try these activities to test your understanding.

Knowledge and Understanding

1) Explain one way that people's ideas about the causes of disease stayed the same between the medieval period and the Renaissance period.

2) Explain why the Church didn't have as much control over medical teaching during the Renaissance as it did in the medieval period.

3) Copy and complete the table below about the work of Vesalius.

	Vesalius' work
a) Methods used to carry out research	
b) Important ideas and discoveries	
c) Important books	
d) Influence on medicine	

Thinking Historically

1) Copy and complete the diagram below. Describe how each aspect of medicine changed during Vesalius' lifetime, and explain whether each change was due to the influence of Vesalius, shifting attitudes in society, technological developments or a combination of these factors.

The medieval period   Vesalius' lifetime

| Dissection was outlawed by the Catholic Church. | → | a) Change: | → | b) Reason for change: |

| There was no easy way to spread new medical ideas. | → | c) Change: | → | d) Reason for change: |

| The teachings of Galen were accepted without question. | → | e) Change: | → | f) Reason for change: |

EXAM TIP

The Renaissance was an age of new ideas...

It really helps to add some important facts in your answers — a useful date, for example. But make sure they're relevant — the details should be used to support your argument.

The Renaissance

<u>William Harvey</u> and <u>Ambroise Paré</u> were key individuals in the history of <u>Renaissance medicine</u>. Harvey discovered how blood <u>circulates</u> around the body, and Paré made surgery <u>safer</u> and <u>more effective</u>.

Harvey discovered the Circulation of the Blood

1) <u>William Harvey</u> was a British doctor, born in <u>1578</u>. He studied medicine at <u>Padua University</u>, Italy, then worked in London at the <u>Royal College of Physicians</u> (see p.28), before becoming <u>Royal Physician</u> to James I and Charles I.

> Harvey was one of many British doctors who studied medicine at a <u>university</u> in <u>Italy</u> or <u>France</u>. During the Renaissance, major <u>new discoveries</u> were being made at these <u>European universities</u> — the discoveries of <u>Vesalius</u> (see p.22) were made at <u>Padua University</u>. British doctors who studied in Europe learnt the <u>latest ideas</u> in medicine and brought them back to <u>Britain</u>.

2) Harvey studied both <u>animals</u> and <u>humans</u> for his work. He realised that he could <u>observe</u> living <u>animal</u> hearts in action, and that his findings would also apply to <u>humans</u>.

3) Before Harvey, people thought that there were <u>two kinds</u> of <u>blood</u>, and that they flowed through two <u>completely separate</u> systems of blood vessels. This idea came from <u>Galen</u>.

A diagram from Harvey's book 'On the Motions of the Heart and Blood' (1628), showing blood circulation in the arm.

4) Harvey realised Galen's theory was <u>wrong</u>. From experiments, he knew that <u>too much</u> blood was being pumped out of the heart for it to be continually formed and consumed. Instead he thought that blood must <u>circulate</u> — it went <u>round and round</u> the body.

5) Harvey's ideas, shown in his books, gave doctors a <u>map</u> of how the <u>body</u> worked, changing their understanding of <u>anatomy</u>.

6) However, not everyone <u>believed</u> his theories, and it took a long time before doctors used them in their <u>treatments</u>. For example, people continued to perform <u>bloodletting</u> (see p.12), even though Harvey had shown the reasoning behind it to be <u>wrong</u>.

Paré improved Surgical Techniques

1) <u>Ambroise Paré</u> was a French barber-surgeon born in <u>1510</u>. Surgery was still a <u>low status</u> profession. Paré worked for a <u>public hospital</u>, then became an <u>army surgeon</u>.

> Paré also designed quite sophisticated <u>artificial limbs</u>.

2) As an army surgeon, Paré treated many <u>serious injuries</u> caused by <u>war</u>. His experience treating these wounds led him to develop some <u>improved surgical techniques</u>.

- At this time, <u>gunshot wounds</u> often became <u>infected</u>. Doctors didn't understand <u>why</u> this happened or how to <u>treat</u> it. The usual treatment was to <u>burn</u> the wound with a <u>red hot iron</u>, or to pour <u>boiling oil</u> onto it. This may have worked in some cases, but it often did more harm than good.

> A <u>cool salve</u> is a type of ointment.

- During one battle, Paré <u>ran out</u> of oil and resorted, by chance, to a simple <u>cool salve</u> instead. To his surprise the patients treated in this way did <u>better</u> than the ones scalded with oil.

- Paré also improved the treatment of <u>amputations</u>. Before Paré, the severed <u>blood vessels</u> left by amputation were sealed by burning their ends with a <u>red hot iron</u> (cauterisation). Paré invented a method of tying off the vessels with <u>threads</u> (ligatures). This was <u>less painful</u> than cauterisation, so it reduced the chances of the patient dying of <u>shock</u>. However, it did increase the risk of <u>infection</u>.

> Paré's ideas were <u>resisted</u> by doctors who felt that a <u>lowly surgeon</u> shouldn't be listened to. He eventually became surgeon to the <u>King of France</u>, and it was only with the <u>King's support</u> that his ideas started to be accepted.

3) Paré <u>published</u> his ideas to enable other doctors to read about them — <u>British surgeons</u> used the methods of Paré and took inspiration from his work. Over time, his ideas helped <u>improve</u> surgical techniques.

The Renaissance

Harvey and Paré made some important discoveries, but not everyone accepted their findings at first. Try these activities to make sure you understand Harvey and Paré's impact on Renaissance medicine.

Knowledge and Understanding

1) In your own words, explain what people believed about blood before William Harvey made his discoveries.

2) How did William Harvey's work change ideas about blood?

3) Explain how Ambroise Paré improved treatment of the following:

   a) Gunshot wounds   b) Amputations

Thinking Historically

1) Explain how William Harvey's work developed the work of Vesalius. You can use the information on page 22 to help you.

2) Using the boxes below, explain the impact that William Harvey had on medicine in the Renaissance period.

   Methods used to carry out research   Ideas about anatomy   Attitudes towards dissection

3) Copy and complete the table below, giving the similarities and differences between Hugh and Theodoric of Lucca's work, and Paré's work. Use the information on page 14 to help you.

Similarities	Differences

4) Why do you think changes in medicine happened slowly in the period c.1500-c.1700? Explain your answer.

5) Do you think the work of Vesalius, Harvey or Paré was the most important for the development of medicine in the Renaissance period? Explain your answer.

Use the information on pages 22 and 24 to help you.

The circulation of the blood goes round and round...

Don't forget to make sure your spelling, punctuation and grammar are all accurate — there are four marks available for this in the long essay question at the end of the exam.

Treatments: Continuity and Change

Medical treatment <u>improved</u> in the Renaissance. But <u>traditional treatments</u> continued to be popular among <u>ordinary people</u>. Both these trends were seen in the way people responded to the <u>Great Plague</u>.

People used both Old and New Treatments

1) Many doctors were reluctant to accept that <u>Galen</u> was <u>wrong</u>. This meant that they continued to use similar treatments to the Middle Ages, like <u>bloodletting</u> and <u>purging</u> (see p.12). Doctors tended to focus more on <u>reading books</u> than on <u>treating patients</u>.

2) Doctors were also still very <u>expensive</u>. As a result, most people used <u>other healers</u>, such as apothecaries or barber-surgeons (see p.14), or were treated in the home. <u>Herbs</u> were still the main ingredient in many drugs.

3) <u>Superstition</u> and <u>religion</u> were still important. People thought the <u>King's touch</u> could cure <u>scrofula</u> (a skin disease known as the '<u>King's Evil</u>'). <u>Thousands</u> of people with scrofula are thought to have visited <u>King Charles I</u> (1600-1649) in the hope of being cured.

4) Some people sold medicines that <u>didn't work</u>, and often did more <u>harm</u> than good — this was known as <u>quackery</u>. <u>Quacks</u> sold their wares at fairs and markets and often had <u>no</u> medical knowledge. From 1600 the College of Physicians (see p.28) started to <u>license</u> doctors to <u>stop</u> quackery.

5) In the 1700s, <u>electricity</u> started to be used in some medical treatments, although it was <u>rarely effective</u>.

> ### Comment and Analysis
> The invention of <u>printing</u> in the 1440s was a huge development. But because most people couldn't <u>read</u> or <u>write</u> (or <u>couldn't afford</u> the books in the first place) new ideas could only be shared within a <u>small part</u> of society. Most people in the Renaissance were using the same cures and treatments as <u>medieval</u> people.

Responses to the Great Plague showed Continuity and Change

1) The Great Plague struck London in <u>1665</u> — it was a rare but deadly <u>recurrence</u> of the medieval <u>Black Death</u> (see p.18).

2) Responses to the <u>Great Plague</u> were both <u>similar</u> and <u>different</u> to how people reacted to the <u>Black Death</u>.

Similarities	Differences
• Many treatments for the Great Plague were based on <u>magic</u>, <u>religion</u> and <u>superstition</u>, including wearing <u>lucky charms</u> or <u>amulets</u>, saying <u>prayers</u> and <u>fasting</u>. • <u>Bloodletting</u> was still used, even though this probably made the plague <u>worse</u> — it created wounds which could become infected. • Some people also thought that <u>miasma</u> caused the disease (see p.8), so they carried posies of <u>herbs</u> or <u>flowers</u> to improve the air.	Town and Parish Councils tried to prevent the disease's <u>spread</u>. • Plague victims were <u>quarantined</u> (isolated) to stop them passing on the disease. The victim's house was <u>locked</u> and a <u>red cross</u> was painted on their door. • Areas where people <u>crowded</u> together, such as <u>theatres</u>, were <u>closed</u>. • The dead bodies of plague victims were buried in <u>mass graves</u> away from houses.

3) The responses to the plague came from <u>local councils</u> — they did more to try to combat the Great Plague than they had done for the Black Death 300 years previously. But there were <u>no national government</u> attempts at prevention.

4) The plague gradually began to <u>disappear</u>. Many people think the <u>Great Fire of London</u> in 1666 helped <u>wipe it out</u>, by effectively <u>sterilising</u> large parts of London — it burned down the <u>old</u>, <u>crowded houses</u>, killing the plague <u>bacteria</u>.

Treatments: Continuity and Change

Although there was some progress in treatments during the Renaissance, some treatments stayed the same. This page will help you understand some examples of continuity and change during this period.

Knowledge and Understanding

1) Give two similarities between doctors in the Renaissance period and doctors in the Middle Ages.

2) Give an example which shows that superstition was still important in the treatment of disease during the first half of the 17th century.

3) What was a quack? Give as much detail as possible.

4) In your own words, describe three ways that local councils tried to stop the Great Plague from spreading.

5) The boxes below contain two different theories about the causes of disease. Write down the responses to the Great Plague that were based on each theory.

a) The miasma theory

b) The Theory of the Four Humours

Thinking Historically

1) Copy and complete the table below, ticking the relevant box to show whether each factor caused continuity, change or both to medicine between the Middle Ages and the Renaissance period. Give an explanation for each choice, using the information from pages 18-26 to help you.

Factor	Continuity	Change	Both
a) **Communication**			
b) **Religion**			
c) **Local government**			

2) Explain why responses to the Great Plague were no more effective than responses to the Black Death. Use the headings in the boxes below to help you write your answer.

You can use information from pages 18 and 26 to help you answer question 2.

Ideas about the cause of disease

Methods of treatment

EXAM TIP

Visiting a quack doctor wasn't usually very produck-tive...

Understanding how factors like religion and communication caused continuity or change is important — in the exam you'll be asked to assess how different factors affected medicine.

Doctors and Surgery

Over time, doctors started to have more training, and surgeons became more important. John Hunter was a surgeon who established a better approach to surgery, based on learning and experimentation.

Doctors' Training and Knowledge began to Improve

1) Many doctors in Britain trained at the College of Physicians, which was set up in 1518. Here they read books by Galen, but also studied recent medical developments. Doctors who trained at the college gained a licence, which separated them from the large numbers of quack doctors (see p.26).

2) However, a licence didn't guarantee that a doctor would give the most effective treatment — sometimes an experienced, unlicensed doctor could be just as good.

3) New weapons like cannons and guns were used in war. This meant surgeons had to treat injuries they hadn't seen before, forcing them to quickly find new treatments.

4) Explorations abroad brought new ingredients for drugs back to Britain, including guaiacum — believed to cure syphilis — and quinine, a drug for malaria from the bark of the Cinchona tree. Other exotic drugs that were sold might have just been advertising gimmicks.

5) Dissections, which enable doctors to see how the body actually works, became a key part of medical training in the 1700s.

> The College of Physicians was later called the Royal College of Physicians.

Surgeons became more Important

1) In the Middle Ages, there were two types of surgeons. There was a small group of professional surgeons, who trained at university and were highly paid by their rich patients. Then there were unqualified barber-surgeons (see p.14). In general, surgeons weren't respected compared to doctors.

2) In the 1700s and 1800s, surgeons began to gain the same status as doctors. In 1800, the London College of Surgeons (later the Royal College of Surgeons) was created, which set training standards for surgeons for the first time.

John Hunter developed Better Approaches to Surgery

John Hunter (1728-93) was a well-known surgeon and scientist.

1) Hunter joined his brother William, a successful doctor, at his anatomy school in London. Dissecting human corpses was a large part of the school's teaching. Over 12 years, Hunter was present at more than 2000 dissections, developing an unrivalled knowledge of the human body.

2) Hunter became an army surgeon in France and Portugal and a popular surgeon and teacher in England. During his work, he made several important medical discoveries. He learned more about venereal disease (sexually transmitted infection), a major cause of illness at the time, and introduced a new approach to the treatment of gunshot wounds.

3) In an operation in 1785, he introduced a new way to treat an aneurysm (a bulge in a blood vessel) in a man's thigh. Hunter tied off the blood vessel to encourage the blood to flow through the other vessels in the leg, preventing it from having to be amputated.

4) Hunter is especially remembered for encouraging better approaches to surgery. This included good scientific habits like learning as much about the body as possible to understand illness, experimenting to find better ways to treat disease, and testing treatments (e.g. on animals) before using them on people.

Comment and Analysis

Hunter's pupils included doctors like Edward Jenner (see p.32). This meant that his methods and ideas were passed on, improving the way people conducted scientific research as a whole.

Doctors and Surgery

Complete these activities to make sure you understand the developments in surgery and doctors' training.

Knowledge and Understanding

1) Explain how overseas exploration affected medical treatments.

2) Copy and complete the mind map below, giving different reasons why doctors' training and knowledge improved in the Renaissance period.

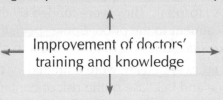

Improvement of doctors' training and knowledge

Thinking Historically

1) Explain how each of the factors below affected surgery in the period c.1500-c.1800. Use the information on pages 22, 24 and 28 to help you.

a) War   b) Individuals   c) Communication   d) Institutions

2) Which of the factors above do you think was the most important in the development of surgery in the period c.1500-c.1800? Explain your answer.

Source Analysis

The source below is from the introduction to a book written by John Hunter in 1793. In the source, Hunter is recalling his time as an army surgeon.

> [This] gave me extensive opportunities of attending to gunshot wounds, of seeing the errors and defects in that branch of military surgery, and of studying to remove them. It drew my attention to inflammation in general, and enabled me to make observations which have formed the basis of the present Treatise*... The object of this book is the improvement of surgery in general, and particularly of that branch of it which is peculiarly directed to the service of the army.

*book

1) Imagine that you are using this source for an investigation into surgery in the 1700s. Explain how the features of the source below affect its usefulness for your investigation.

a) Author   b) Content   c) Purpose

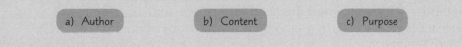

The Beginnings of Change

Hospitals

From the 18th century, hospitals focused more on <u>treating</u> patients — rather than just <u>caring</u> for them — as well as <u>teaching</u>. <u>Nursing</u> standards also improved — largely thanks to <u>Florence Nightingale</u>.

Hospitals focused more on Treatment and Learning

In the <u>1530s</u>, Henry VIII closed down most of Britain's <u>monasteries</u> (this was called the '<u>dissolution of the monasteries</u>'). Since most hospitals had been set up and run by monasteries (see p.16), this also led to the <u>closure</u> of a large number of <u>hospitals</u>. As a result, Britain had relatively <u>few hospitals</u> until the 18th century.

1) From the early 18th century, several <u>charity hospitals</u> opened, including the Middlesex Infirmary, The London Hospital and Guy's Hospital. They were funded by the <u>rich</u>, and offered <u>largely free</u> treatment to the poor. Some <u>specialised</u> in treating certain illnesses, or provided somewhere for mothers to <u>give birth</u>.

Comment and Analysis

Before the 18th century, many hospitals focused only on <u>caring</u> for people. In the 18th and 19th centuries, <u>treating</u> diseases became more important.

2) Only those who were likely to <u>recover quickly</u> were admitted — this was partly because of a <u>lack of space</u> and because of the risk of contagious illnesses <u>spreading</u>. The '<u>deserving</u>' poor (those who led hardworking, respectable lives) had a greater chance of being admitted.

3) <u>Dispensaries</u> provided <u>free non-residential care</u> to poor people. <u>Medicines</u> and <u>non-surgical</u> services from people like <u>dentists</u> and <u>midwives</u> were given without charge.

4) Most poor people were treated in <u>workhouses</u> — large buildings that people went to if they could no longer look after themselves (e.g. because of unemployment, illness or old age). <u>Conditions</u> were <u>poor</u> — from the 1850s a partially successful movement began to <u>improve conditions</u> in <u>workhouse infirmaries</u>.

5) In the 19th century, some hospitals were founded alongside <u>universities</u> or <u>medical schools</u>, including Charing Cross Hospital, University College Hospital and King's College Hospital. These hospitals were used as <u>training schools</u> for doctors, and for conducting <u>scientific research</u>.

6) <u>Cottage hospitals</u>, run by <u>GPs</u>, opened from the 1860s. They provided care for people in <u>rural</u> areas.

Florence Nightingale Improved Nursing Standards

1) Florence Nightingale (1820-1910) studied to become a nurse in 1849, despite opposition from her family. During her career, she helped nursing become more <u>professional</u> and <u>disciplined</u>.

2) When the <u>Crimean War</u> broke out in 1853-54, horror stories emerged about the Barrack Hospital in <u>Scutari</u>, where the British wounded were treated. <u>Sidney Herbert</u> (the Secretary of War and a friend of her family) asked for Nightingale to go to Scutari to sort out the <u>nursing care</u> in the hospital.

3) The army <u>opposed</u> women nurses, as they were considered inferior and a distraction. Nightingale went anyway, taking <u>38 hand-picked nurses</u> with her.

4) Using methods she had learned from her training in Europe, Nightingale ensured all the wards were <u>clean</u> and <u>hygienic</u>, that water supplies were adequate and that patients were fed properly.

Nightingale <u>improved</u> the hospital a lot. Before she arrived, the <u>death rate</u> in the hospital stood at <u>42%</u>. Two years later it had fallen to just <u>2%</u>.

5) Many of Nightingale's nursing practices were used in hospitals in <u>Britain</u>.

- In 1859, Nightingale published a book, '<u>Notes on Nursing</u>'. This explained her methods — it emphasised the need for <u>hygiene</u> and a <u>professional attitude</u>. It was the <u>standard textbook</u> for generations of nurses.

- The public raised <u>£44,000</u> to help her <u>train nurses</u>, and she set up the <u>Nightingale School of Nursing</u> in St. Thomas' Hospital, London. Nurses were given <u>three years</u> of training before they could qualify. <u>Discipline</u> and <u>attention to detail</u> were important.

Hospitals

These activities will help you understand how hospitals and nursing improved in the period c.1700-c.1900.

Knowledge and Understanding

1) Describe the following places that provided medical treatment in the 18th and 19th centuries:

a) charity hospitals   b) dispensaries   c) workhouses   d) medical school hospitals   e) cottage hospitals

Thinking Historically

1) Copy and complete the table below, comparing hospitals in medieval England (p.14) and hospitals in the period c.1700-c.1900.

Aspect of hospital	Medieval hospitals	Hospitals in c.1700-c.1900
a) Number of hospitals		
b) Who ran them?		
c) Their purpose		
d) Cleanliness		

Source Analysis

The source below was published in 1856. It shows a ward at Scutari Hospital, a war hospital in Crimea. Florence Nightingale is shown in black on the left talking to an army officer.

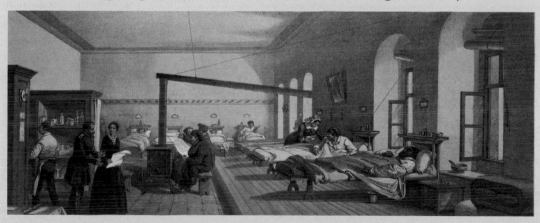

1) What does this source suggest about Florence Nightingale's influence on nursing? Use details from the source to support you answer.

2) The source was drawn by an artist who visited Crimea during the war there. How does this affect the usefulness of the source for studying the development of hospitals in the 19th century?

EXAM TIP

Don't Crimea river — just learn the stuff on this page...

As well as learning and understanding the key achievements of individuals like Florence Nightingale, you also need to be able to explain why their work was significant.

Jenner and Vaccination

Until the 1700s, people had <u>few</u> effective ways to <u>prevent</u> the spread of <u>disease</u>. <u>Edward Jenner's</u> discovery of the <u>smallpox vaccine</u> was a <u>landmark</u> in the development of <u>preventive medicine</u>.

Before Jenner the only way to prevent Smallpox was Inoculation

1) In the 1700s, <u>smallpox</u> was one of the most <u>deadly</u> diseases — in 1751, over 3500 people died of smallpox in London alone.

2) At the time, the only way to prevent smallpox was <u>inoculation</u>. This was promoted in Britain by Lady Mary Wortley Montagu, who learned about it in Turkey.

3) Inoculation involved making a <u>cut</u> in a patient's arm and soaking it in pus taken from the swelling of somebody who already had a <u>mild form</u> of smallpox.

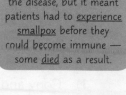

Inoculation was successful in preventing the disease, but it meant patients had to <u>experience</u> <u>smallpox</u> before they could become immune — some <u>died</u> as a result.

Jenner discovered a link between Smallpox and Cowpox

1) <u>Edward Jenner</u> (born in 1749) was a country doctor in <u>Gloucestershire</u>. He heard that <u>milkmaids</u> didn't get smallpox, but they did catch the much milder <u>cowpox</u>.

2) Using careful <u>scientific methods</u> Jenner investigated and discovered that it was true that people who had had <u>cowpox</u> didn't get <u>smallpox</u>.

3) In 1796 Jenner <u>tested</u> his theory. He injected a small boy, <u>James Phipps</u>, with pus from the sores of <u>Sarah Nelmes</u>, a milkmaid with cowpox. Jenner then infected him with smallpox. James <u>didn't catch</u> the disease.

4) Jenner <u>published</u> his findings in <u>1798</u>. He coined the term vaccination using the Latin word for cow, <u>vacca</u>.

Comment and Analysis

Jenner was important because he used an <u>experiment</u> to test his theory. Although experiments had been used during the Renaissance, it was still <u>unusual</u> for doctors to <u>test</u> their theories.

Jenner's vaccination was Successful despite Opposition

1) Jenner faced some <u>opposition</u> to his vaccine...

- Many people were <u>worried</u> about giving themselves a disease from <u>cows</u>.

- Some <u>doctors</u> who gave the older type of inoculation saw it as a <u>threat</u> to their livelihood.

- One doctor, <u>William Woodville</u>, claimed Jenner's vaccination worked little better than inoculation, after several smallpox deaths occurred at his hospital.

- When vaccination became <u>compulsory</u> in 1853, several groups were formed to <u>campaign</u> <u>against it</u> — they didn't like the idea of the <u>government</u> telling them what to do.

2) ...but his discovery got the approval of <u>Parliament</u>.

- In 1802, Parliament gave Jenner <u>£10,000</u> to open a vaccination clinic. It gave Jenner a further <u>£20,000</u> a few years later.

- In 1840, vaccination against smallpox was made <u>free</u> for infants. In 1853, it was made <u>compulsory</u>.

- The vaccine was a <u>success</u> — it contributed to a big fall in the number of smallpox cases in Britain.

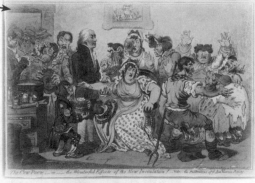

A cartoon from 1802 by James Gillray, with cows bursting out of vaccinated patients' sores.

© Mary Evans Picture Library

Comment and Analysis

Jenner <u>didn't know</u> why his vaccine worked. This <u>lack of understanding</u> meant Jenner <u>couldn't</u> develop any other vaccines. This was only possible after the Germ Theory was published in 1861, when <u>Pasteur</u> and others worked to discover vaccines against other diseases, like chicken cholera, anthrax and rabies (see p.36-38).

Jenner and Vaccination

SKILLS PRACTICE

Have a go at these activities to test your knowledge of the development of Jenner's smallpox vaccine.

Knowledge and Understanding

1) Explain how smallpox was prevented before Jenner developed his vaccination. Include the following key words in your explanation.

cut   inoculation   patient's arm

2) Explain why Jenner's smallpox vaccine was safer than the smallpox inoculation.

3) Copy and complete the timeline below about the decline of smallpox in Britain. Fill in all the key events between 1796 and 1853, and include as much detail as you can.

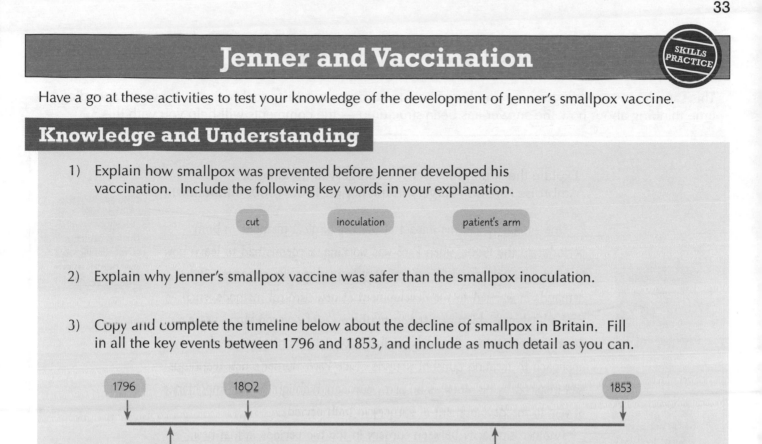

1796   1802   1853

1798   1840

Thinking Historically

1) Explain why social attitudes led to some opposition to Jenner's vaccination.

2) Copy and complete the mind map below, giving examples of the role Parliament and individuals played in the development of the smallpox vaccination.

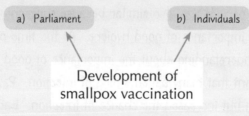

a) Parliament   b) Individuals

Development of smallpox vaccination

3) Do you think Parliament or individuals were more important to the success of the smallpox vaccination? Explain your answer.

4) Explain the similarities between Jenner's development of the smallpox vaccination and Harvey's work on the circulation of blood (see p.24). You should discuss the following points:

Research methods   Development of existing ideas   Response to findings

EXAM TIP

Jenner's vaccine got disease prevention mooving...

Remember to use linking words and phrases like 'however', 'because of this', 'as a result' and 'therefore' to clearly show the link between an event and its causes and consequences.

The Beginnings of Change

Worked Exam-Style Question

This sample answer will give you an idea of how to compare two historical periods. It's worth spending time thinking about how the answer has been structured — the comments will help you with this.

Explain the similarities between surgery at the time of
Ambroise Paré and surgery in the period 1700-1900.   [8 marks]

> This addresses the question in the first sentence by mentioning an important feature of both periods.

One similarity was the impact of war on surgical methods in both periods. In the 1500s, when Paré was working, surgeons had to learn how to treat injuries caused by new military technology like cannons. The demands of war led to the development of new surgical methods, such as Paré's ligatures, which he used to tie the ends of severed blood vessels during amputations. Similarly, in the 1700s John Hunter invented a new approach to treating gunshot wounds. Like Paré, Hunter's new technique was inspired by his work as an army surgeon, highlighting the importance of war to the development of surgery in both periods.

> Using specific information shows good knowledge of the period.

> To get a high mark, you need to give more than one similarity.

> Use words like 'similarly' to show that you are comparing.

Another similarity between surgery in the two periods is that new surgical ideas could take a long time to make an impact. Even though Paré published his work, many doctors refused to take his innovations seriously — it was only once he became the French king's surgeon that his ideas gained recognition. Similarly, in the period 1700-1900 surgeons were slow to adopt new ideas such as anaesthetics. As early as 1799, Humphry Davy identified nitrous oxide as a possible anaesthetic, but his findings were ignored. Anaesthetics only began to be widely used in surgery over fifty years later, after Queen Victoria gave birth to her eighth child using chloroform in 1853.

> Make sure you include plenty of specific, relevant information, such as key dates and figures.

Surgery in both periods was also similar because surgeons did not understand the importance of good hygiene. At the time of Paré, surgeons' lack of understanding about the importance of good hygiene while operating meant that many patients died of infection. Paré's ligatures eased pain but increased the chance of infection. Lack of understanding about hygiene was also a problem for much of the period 1700-1900. In the 1860s, surgeons were still working in dirty clothes and were reluctant to wash their hands with chloride of lime between operations, as they found it too unpleasant. It was only in the years after the publication of Pasteur's Germ Theory in 1861 that surgeons began to understand the importance of good hygiene. The introduction of Joseph Lister's carbolic spray in the 1860s reduced infection, and hygiene improved even further with the development of aseptic surgical methods from the late 19th century. However, for most of the period 1700-1900, surgical hygiene was as poor as it was in the time of Paré.

> Comparing the two periods in every point you make shows your answer is focused on the question.

> Use wider knowledge of the period to support your argument.

The Beginnings of Change

Exam-Style Questions

Answer the questions below to make sure you understand what you've learnt about medicine in this section.

Source A

A cartoon produced in 1802. It shows Edward Jenner and two other doctors pouring infants into a cow-like creature's mouth. The infants are excreted by the creature with horns and tails. The creature is covered in sores and names of other diseases such as 'Plague' and 'Leprosy'. In Jenner's back pocket is a document with the figure '£10,000' written on it.

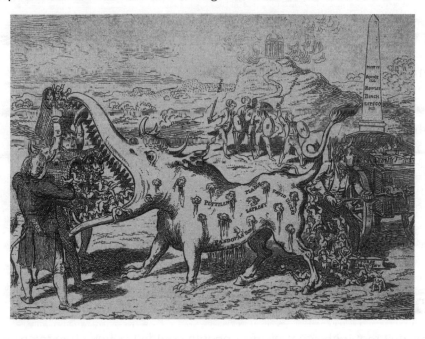

Exam-Style Questions

1) Look at Source A. How useful would it be for an investigation into Jenner's work on vaccination? Use Source A and your own knowledge to explain your answer. [8 marks]

2) Explain why the work of William Harvey was important for the development of medicine. [8 marks]

3) Explain the similarities between the Black Death in the Middle Ages and the Great Plague in the 17th century. [8 marks]

4) Has the role of individuals been the most important factor in understanding the causes of disease since the Middle Ages? Explain your answer.

> For the 16-mark question in the exam, 4 extra marks will be available for spelling, punctuation, grammar and using specialist terminology.

Your answer should discuss the role of individuals and other factors. Make sure you include examples from across the period c.1000 to the present day. [16 marks]

A Revolution in Medicine

The Germ Theory

Although people's understanding of <u>anatomy</u> had improved greatly during the Renaissance, there was still plenty to learn. The <u>causes of disease</u> was an area that still needed proper explanation.

People knew about Germs but hadn't linked them to Disease

Germs and other <u>micro-organisms</u> were discovered as early as the 17th century. Scientists thought that these microbes were <u>created</u> by <u>decaying matter</u>, like rotting food or human waste — this theory was known as <u>spontaneous generation</u>. It led people to believe that <u>disease caused germs</u>.

Pasteur was the first to suggest that Germs cause disease

1) The French chemist <u>Louis Pasteur</u> was employed in <u>1857</u> to find the explanation for the <u>souring</u> of sugar beet used in fermenting industrial <u>alcohol</u>. His answer was to blame <u>germs</u>.

2) Pasteur proved there were germs in the air — he showed that sterilised water in a closed flask <u>stayed sterile</u>, while sterilised water in an open flask <u>bred germs</u>.

3) In <u>1861</u>, Pasteur published his <u>Germ Theory</u>. In it he argued that <u>microbes</u> in the air <u>caused decay</u>, not the other way round. He also suggested that some <u>germs caused disease</u>.

4) In 1867, Pasteur published evidence <u>proving</u> there was a link between germs and disease, demonstrating that germs caused a disease in <u>silkworms</u>.

> Pasteur's discovery was partly due to Antonie <u>van Leeuwenhoek's</u> invention of the <u>microscope</u> in the 17th century. <u>More advanced microscopes</u> were developed during the 1800s. They allowed scientists to see much <u>clearer images</u> with a lot <u>less light distortion</u>.

The Germ Theory had a major Impact on medicine

The Germ Theory was first met with <u>scepticism</u> — people <u>couldn't believe</u> tiny microbes caused disease. It didn't help that the germ responsible for each disease had to be identified <u>individually</u>, as this meant it was <u>several years</u> before the theory became useful. Eventually, however, it gained popularity in Britain.

- The theory helped inspire <u>Joseph Lister</u> to develop <u>antiseptics</u> (see p.42).
- The theory confirmed <u>John Snow's</u> findings about <u>cholera</u> (see p.44).
- The theory linked disease to poor living conditions (like contaminated water). This put pressure on the government to pass the <u>1875 Public Health Act</u> (see p.46).

Robert Koch used dyes to identify microbes

1) The German scientist <u>Robert Koch</u> built on Pasteur's work by linking specific diseases to the particular <u>microbe</u> that caused them. This technique was called '<u>microbe hunting</u>'.

2) Koch identified <u>anthrax</u> bacteria (<u>1876</u>) and the bacteria that cause <u>septicaemia</u> (<u>1878</u>), <u>tuberculosis</u> (<u>1882</u>) and <u>cholera</u> (<u>1883</u>).

3) Koch used revolutionary <u>scientific methods</u>:

- He used <u>agar jelly</u> to create solid <u>cultures</u>, allowing him to breed lots of bacteria.
- He used <u>dyes</u> to <u>stain</u> the bacteria so they were more visible under the microscope.
- He employed the newly-invented <u>photography</u> to record his findings.

4) Koch's techniques were important as they allowed other <u>microbe hunters</u> to find the specific bacteria which cause other diseases (see p.38).

The Germ Theory

The Germ Theory had a big impact on understanding diseases — this page will show you its significance.

Knowledge and Understanding

1) Explain the ideas behind each of the following terms:
   a) Spontaneous generation
   b) The Germ Theory

2) In your own words, explain how Pasteur proved there were germs in the air.

3) State the scientific discovery Robert Koch made in each of the following years:

   a) 1876   b) 1878   c) 1882   d) 1883

4) Copy and complete the mind map below, giving examples of new technology and scientific methods which helped Robert Koch to develop his ideas on the causes of disease.

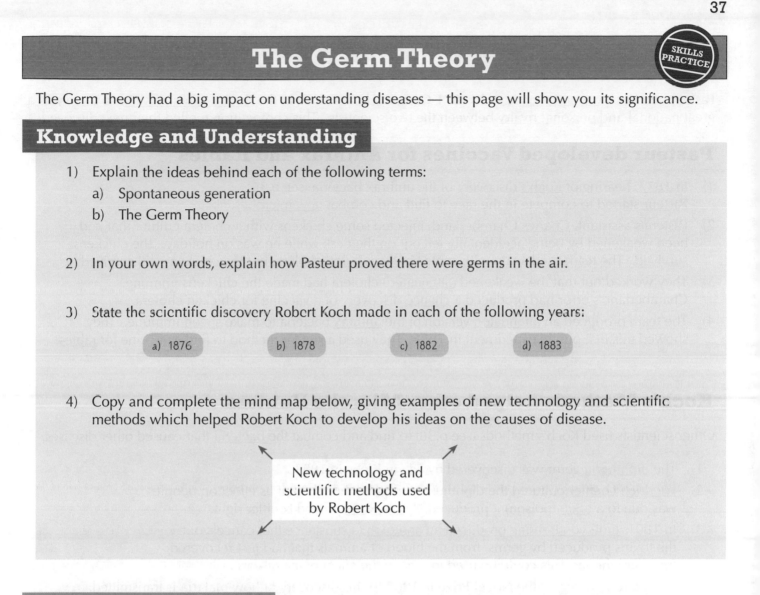

New technology and scientific methods used by Robert Koch

Thinking Historically

1) Do you think the role of individuals or new technology was more important in the development of the Germ Theory? Explain your answer, referring to both factors.

2) The Germ Theory and Jenner's smallpox vaccination were both important breakthroughs. Copy and complete the table below, explaining why each discovery was important for the development of medicine. Use information from pages 32 and 36 to help you.

Discovery	Why it was important for the development of medicine
a) The Germ Theory	
b) Smallpox vaccination	

3) Do you think the Germ Theory or the smallpox vaccination was more important for the development of medicine? Explain your answer, referring to both factors.

EXAM TIP

Pasteur's theory — more than the germ of an idea...

When you're learning about discoveries by scientists like Koch, it's important to think about how developments that came beforehand (like the Germ Theory) made their work possible.

The Fight against Germs

Pasteur and Koch weren't friends — in 1871 Germany beat France in the Franco-Prussian War, so there was a great national and personal rivalry between the two scientists. This competition fuelled their next discoveries.

Pasteur developed Vaccines for Anthrax and Rabies

1) In 1877, hearing of Koch's discovery of the anthrax bacteria (see p.36), Pasteur started to compete in the race to find and combat new microbes.

2) Pasteur's assistant, Charles Chamberland, injected some chickens with a cholera culture that had been weakened by being accidentally left out on the desk while he was on holiday. The chickens survived. The team tried again with some newly cultured cholera, but the chickens still survived.

3) They worked out that the weakened (attenuated) cholera had made the chickens immune. Chamberland's error had produced a chance discovery of a vaccine for chicken cholera.

4) The team produced an attenuated version of the anthrax bacteria to make sheep immune. They showed this in a public experiment in 1881. They used a similar method to find a vaccine for rabies.

Koch's Methods helped other Microbe Hunters

Other scientists used Koch's methods (see p.36) to find and combat the bacteria that caused other diseases.

1) The diphtheria germ was discovered by Edwin Klebs in 1883.

2) Friedrich Loeffler cultured the diphtheria germ and thought that its effect on people was due to a toxin (poison) it produced. Emile Roux proved Loeffler right.

3) In 1891, Emil von Behring produced an antitoxin (a substance that cancels out the toxins produced by germs) from the blood of animals that had just recovered from diphtheria. This could be used to reduce the effect of the disease.

4) Ronald Ross received the Nobel Prize in 1902 for his discovery of how malaria is transmitted. Ross' Nobel Prize was disputed by Giovanni Battista Grassi, who also discovered how malaria is transmitted. However, Koch supported Ross' claim and so he retained the prize.

Paul Ehrlich discovered the first Magic Bullet — Salvarsan 606

Antibodies were identified as a natural defence mechanism of the body against germs. It was known that antibodies only attacked specific microbes — so they were nicknamed magic bullets. In 1889, Paul Ehrlich set out to find chemicals that could act as synthetic antibodies.

1) First, Ehrlich discovered dyes that could kill the malaria and sleeping sickness germs.

2) In 1905, the bacteria that causes the sexually transmitted disease syphilis was identified.

3) Ehrlich and his team decided to search for an arsenic compound that was a magic bullet for syphilis. They hoped it would target the bacteria without poisoning the rest of the body. Over 600 compounds were tried, but none seemed to work.

4) In 1909, Sahachiro Hata joined the team. He rechecked the results and saw that compound number 606 actually appeared to work. It was first used on a human in 1911 under the trade name Salvarsan 606.

Comment and Analysis

The Germ Theory led to the introduction of new vaccines, antiseptics (see p.42) and government intervention in public health (see p.46). But it didn't really affect treatments in Britain that much — Salvarsan 606 was only a treatment for one specific disease, and the second magic bullet (prontosil) wasn't discovered until 1935. It wasn't until the pharmaceutical industry took off in the 1940s (see p.54) that ordinary people began to feel a benefit from the Germ Theory.

The Fight against Germs

More names, more discoveries, more treatments — do these activities to make sure you've got them sussed.

Knowledge and Understanding

1) Give three vaccines that Pasteur's team developed.

2) Describe the discoveries made by each of the following microbe hunters:
    a) Edwin Klebs
    b) Friedrich Loeffler
    c) Emil von Behring
    d) Ronald Ross

3) What is meant by the term 'magic bullet'?

4) Copy and complete the timeline below, summarising the events related to
    the discovery of Salvarsan 606. Try to give as much detail as you can.

1889			1905	1909	1911

Thinking Historically

1) Copy and complete the table below, explaining how each
    factor contributed to the development of new vaccines.

Factor	Contribution to the development of new vaccines
a) Individuals	
b) Chance	

2) Which of the factors in the table above do you think was the most
    important for the development of new vaccines? Explain your answer.

3) Explain why Robert Koch was important for the
    development of medicine in the 19th century.

4) Why was there only slow progress in the treatment
    of disease between the 1860s and the 1940s?

> You can use information
> from pages 36 and 38
> to help you answer
> questions 3 and 4.

When it comes to magic bullets, Ehrlich hit the mark...

*Make sure you know how much time to spend on each question in the exam — if one question
is worth twice as many marks as another, you should spend about twice as long answering it.*

A Revolution in Medicine

Anaesthetics

Improving <u>hospitals</u> helped to prevent many unnecessary deaths. But the three problems of <u>pain</u>, <u>infection</u> (see p.42) and <u>blood loss</u> (see p.50) were yet to be solved. The solution to pain was <u>anaesthetics</u>.

Anaesthetics solved the problem of Pain

Pain was a problem for surgeons, especially since patients could <u>die</u> from the <u>trauma</u> of extreme pain. Natural drugs like <u>alcohol</u>, <u>opium</u> and <u>mandrake</u> had been used for a long time, but effective <u>anaesthetics</u> that didn't make the patient <u>very ill</u> were more difficult to produce.

- <u>Nitrous oxide</u> (laughing gas) was identified as a possible anaesthetic by British chemist <u>Humphry Davy</u> in <u>1799</u> — but he was <u>ignored</u> by surgeons at the time.
- The gas had been dismissed as a fairground novelty before American <u>dentist Horace Wells</u> suggested its use in his area of work. He did a <u>public demonstration</u> in <u>1845</u>, but had the bad luck to pick a patient unaffected by nitrous oxide — it was <u>again ignored</u>.

  - In <u>1842</u>, American doctor <u>Crawford Long</u> discovered the anaesthetic qualities of <u>ether</u>, but didn't publish his work. The first <u>public demonstration</u> of ether as an anaesthetic was carried out in <u>1846</u> by American dental surgeon <u>William Morton</u>.
  - Ether is an <u>irritant</u> and is also fairly <u>explosive</u>, so using it in this way was risky.

    - <u>James Simpson</u> was a Professor of Midwifery at Edinburgh University who tried to find a safe alternative to ether that women could take during <u>childbirth</u>. He began to experiment with <u>other chemicals</u> by testing them on <u>himself</u>.
    - In <u>1847</u> Simpson discovered the effects of <u>chloroform</u>. He found it was <u>easier</u> to use than ether — it took effect <u>more quickly</u> and <u>less was needed</u> to achieve the same result.
    - After <u>Queen Victoria</u> gave birth to her eighth child while using chloroform in 1853, it became <u>widely used</u> in operating theatres and to reduce pain during childbirth.

<u>General anaesthesia</u> (complete unconsciousness) is <u>risky</u>, so <u>local anaesthesia</u> (numbing of the part being treated) is better for many operations. In <u>1884</u>, <u>William Halsted</u> investigated the use of <u>cocaine</u> as a local anaesthetic. His self-experimentation led to a severe cocaine <u>addiction</u>.

Early Anaesthetics actually led to a Rise in death rates

1) Anaesthetics led to <u>longer</u> and <u>more complex</u> operations. This was because surgeons found that unconscious patients were <u>easier to operate on</u>, meaning they could take <u>longer</u> over their work.

2) Longer operating times led to <u>higher death rates</u> from <u>infection</u>, because surgeons didn't know that <u>poor hygiene</u> spread disease. Surgeons used very <u>unhygienic</u> methods:

   - Surgeons didn't know that having <u>clean clothes</u> could save lives. Often they wore the <u>same coats</u> for years, which were <u>covered</u> in <u>dried blood</u> and <u>pus</u> from previous operations.
   - Operations were often carried out in <u>unhygienic conditions</u>, including at the patient's <u>house</u>.
   - <u>Operating instruments</u> also caused infections because they were usually <u>unwashed</u> and <u>dirty</u>.

Comment and Analysis

Anaesthetics helped solve the problem of <u>pain</u>, but patients were still dying from <u>infection</u>. This meant the attempts at more complicated surgery actually led to <u>increased death rates</u> amongst patients. The period between 1846 and 1870 is sometimes known as the '<u>Black Period</u>' of surgery for this reason.

Anaesthetics

There are a lot of names and dates linked to the development of anaesthetics in Britain in the 1800s. To make sure all that information has sunk in, have a go at the activities on this page.

Knowledge and Understanding

1) Why are anaesthetics important during surgery?

2) Make a flashcard for each person below. Put their name on one side and describe their role in the development of anaesthetics on the other.

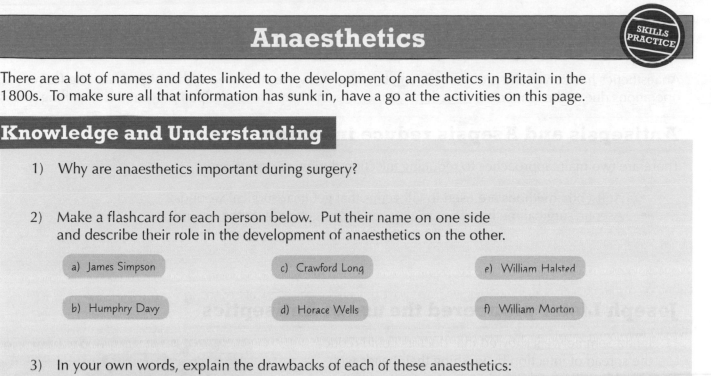

   a) James Simpson   c) Crawford Long   e) William Halsted

   b) Humphry Davy   d) Horace Wells   f) William Morton

3) In your own words, explain the drawbacks of each of these anaesthetics:
   a) Nitrous Oxide (laughing gas)
   b) Ether
   c) Cocaine

4) Why is the period between 1846 and 1870 known as the 'Black Period' of surgery?

Thinking Historically

1) Which individual do you think made the most important contribution to the development of anaesthetics? Explain your answer.

2) How did developments in anaesthetics affect surgery in the short term? Give one positive effect and one negative effect.

3) Copy and complete the table below, explaining whether there was change or continuity in each aspect of surgery between the 1800s and the 1860s.

Aspect of surgery	Change or continuity?	Explanation for choice
a) Clothes worn by surgeons		
b) Use of anaesthetics		
c) Location of surgery		
d) Length of operations		

Anaesthetics revision — don't let it put you to sleep...

In the exam, remember to be specific about the information you use. For instance, rather than writing about anaesthetics in general, try to use specific examples to explain your answer.

A Revolution in Medicine

Antiseptics

Anaesthetics had solved the problem of <u>pain</u>, but surgeons were still faced with a high death rate from operations due to the amount of <u>infection</u>. <u>Antiseptics</u> and later <u>asepsis</u> helped prevent this by killing germs.

Antisepsis and Asepsis reduce infection

There are two main approaches to <u>reducing infection</u> during an operation:

- <u>Antiseptic</u> methods are used to <u>kill germs</u> that get near surgical wounds.
- <u>Aseptic</u> surgical methods aim to <u>stop any germs</u> getting near the wound.

Joseph Lister pioneered the use of Antiseptics

1) <u>Ignaz Semmelweis</u> showed that doctors could reduce the spread of infection by washing their hands with <u>chloride of lime</u> solution between patients. However, it was very <u>unpleasant</u>, so wasn't widely used.

2) <u>Joseph Lister</u> had seen <u>carbolic acid</u> sprays used in <u>sewage works</u> to keep down the smell. He tried this in the operating theatre in the early 1860s and saw reduced infection rates.

3) Lister heard about the <u>Germ Theory</u> in 1865 — he realised that germs could be in the air, on surgical instruments and on people's hands. He started using carbolic acid on <u>instruments</u> and <u>bandages</u>.

4) The use of <u>antiseptics</u> immediately <u>reduced death rates</u> from as high as 50% in 1864-66 to around 15% in 1867-70.

5) Despite these early successes, Lister faced <u>opposition</u> from many doctors. They didn't like to use the carbolic spray, which they found <u>unpleasant</u> on their skin or to breathe in.

6) In 1877, Lister used a well-publicised operation at King's College Hospital to <u>promote</u> the use of his <u>carbolic spray</u>.

7) Antiseptics allowed surgeons to operate with less fear of patients dying from infection. The <u>number of operations</u> was ten times higher in 1912 than 1867 as a result.

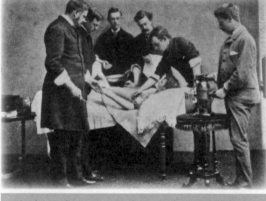

© Mary Evans Picture Library

A photo of an operation from the late 1800s. You can see Lister's <u>carbolic spray</u> on the table on the right. The operating theatre <u>isn't aseptic</u> though — the surgeons aren't wearing sterile gowns or surgical gloves.

Comment and Analysis

Antiseptics (and later asepsis) solved the problem of <u>infection</u>. This, combined with the use of <u>anaesthetics</u> (see p.40) to stop pain, improved British surgery and prevented many deaths.

Asepsis reduced the need for Nasty Chemicals

Since the late 1800s, surgeons have changed their approach from <u>killing germs</u> to making a <u>germ-free</u> (aseptic) environment. Aseptic surgery <u>reduced</u> the need for a carbolic spray.

1) Instruments are carefully <u>sterilised</u> before use, usually with high temperature steam (<u>120°C</u>).

2) Theatre staff <u>sterilise their hands</u> before entering — and wear sterile gowns, masks, gloves and hats. Surgical <u>gloves</u> were invented by <u>William Halsted</u> in <u>1889</u>.

3) The theatres themselves are kept <u>extremely clean</u> and fed with <u>sterile air</u>. Special tents can be placed around the operating table to maintain an area of even stricter hygiene in <u>high risk</u> cases.

Antiseptics

SKILLS PRACTICE

The introduction of antiseptics and asepsis prevented infections and greatly improved British surgery. Try out the activities below to make sure you understand the effect of these developments.

Knowledge and Understanding

1) In your own words, describe the difference between antiseptic and aseptic surgical methods.

2) How did the following contribute to the development of antiseptics?

    a) Ignaz Semmelweis   b) sewage works   c) the Germ Theory

3) What was the main drawback of using carbolic acid during surgery?

4) How do surgeons create an aseptic environment?

Thinking Historically

1) Complete the mind map below, explaining the effect that antiseptics had on surgery in the 19th century. Give as much detail as possible.

← Antiseptics →

↓

2) Which of the factors below do you think was the most important in the development of surgery in the period c.1800-c.1900? Explain your answer.

    individuals   chance   communication

You should refer to all three factors in your answer. Use pages 40-42 to help you.

Source Analysis

The source on the right is a drawing of a surgeon performing an operation. It was published in 1882.

1) How does the date of this source affect its usefulness for studying surgery in the 19th century?

Use pages 40-42 to help you answer both questions.

2) How useful is the content of this source for studying surgery in the 19th century. Explain your answer, using the details in the blue boxes to help you.

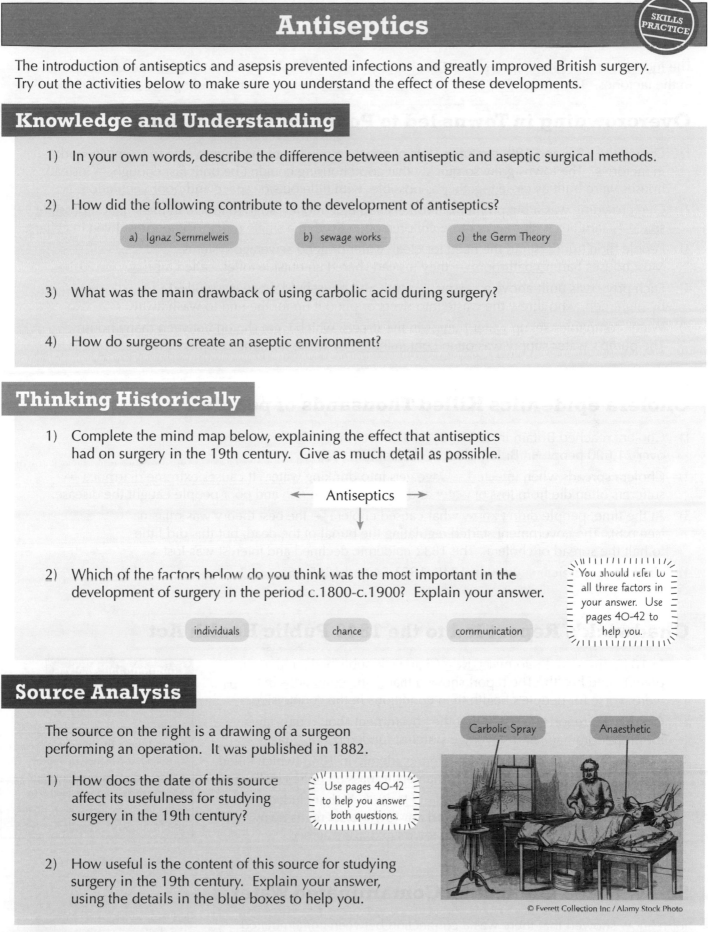

Carbolic Spray   Anaesthetic

© Everett Collection Inc / Alamy Stock Photo

EXAM TIP

Make a Lister them facts — then germ up on them...

You need to be confident about how surgery changed over time. Surgeons started by killing germs with antiseptic methods, and then began to stop germs using aseptic methods as well.

Public Health

The <u>industrial revolution</u> began in the 18th century. Lots of people moved into <u>cities</u> like London to work in the factories. The places they lived were <u>cramped</u>, <u>dirty</u> and great for spreading <u>diseases</u> like cholera.

Overcrowding in Towns led to Poor Living Conditions

1) During the 18th and 19th centuries, lots of people <u>moved</u> from the countryside to <u>towns</u> to work in factories. The towns grew so <u>quickly</u> that good housing couldn't be built fast enough — instead, houses were built as <u>close together</u> as possible, with <u>little outside space</u> and <u>poor ventilation</u>.

2) <u>Overcrowding</u> was a big problem. Workers had little money, so tried to live in the <u>smallest possible space</u> — families with four or more children often lived in a <u>single room</u>. The poorest lived in <u>cellars</u>.

3) People <u>didn't understand</u> the need for clean water or good sewerage systems. Most houses had <u>no bathroom</u> — they instead shared an outside toilet, called a <u>privy</u>.

4) Each privy was built above a <u>cesspit</u>. Cesspit and household waste was collected by <u>nightmen</u>, who threw the waste into rivers or piled it up for the rain to wash away.

5) Water companies set up <u>water pumps</u> in the streets, which were <u>shared</u> between many houses. The pump's water supply was often <u>contaminated</u> by waste from the cesspits or rivers.

Cholera epidemics Killed Thousands of people

1) <u>Cholera</u> reached Britain in 1831. By 1832 it was an <u>epidemic</u> — over 21,000 people in Britain died of cholera that year.

2) Cholera spreads when <u>infected sewage</u> gets into drinking water. It causes extreme <u>diarrhoea</u> — sufferers often die from <u>loss of water</u> and <u>minerals</u>. Both <u>rich</u> and <u>poor</u> people caught the disease.

3) At the time, people <u>didn't know</u> what caused cholera — the best theory was <u>miasma</u> (see p.8). The government started regulating the burial of the dead, but this did little to halt the spread of cholera. The 1832 epidemic declined and interest was lost.

4) Cholera epidemics <u>recurred</u> in 1848, 1853-54 and 1865-66.

Chadwick's Report led to the 1848 Public Health Act

1) In 1842, the social reformer <u>Edwin Chadwick</u> published a report on poverty and health. The report showed that <u>living conditions</u> in <u>towns</u> were <u>worse</u> for people's health than conditions in the <u>countryside</u>.

2) Chadwick's report <u>suggested</u> that the government should <u>pass laws</u> for proper <u>drainage</u> and <u>sewerage</u> systems, funded by <u>local taxes</u>.

3) Chadwick's report and another <u>cholera epidemic</u> in <u>1848</u> (which killed 53,000 people) put <u>pressure</u> on Parliament to pass a <u>Public Health Act</u>.

4) The 1848 Act set up a central <u>Board of Health</u> (which included Chadwick as a member) and allowed any <u>town</u> to set up its own <u>local board of health</u> as long as the town's <u>taxpayers</u> agreed.

Comment and Analysis

The impact of the 1848 Act was <u>limited</u> — towns <u>could</u> set up health boards but <u>very few chose to</u>, and those that did often <u>refused</u> to spend any money to improve conditions. Chadwick <u>annoyed</u> a lot of people, and was forced to retire in 1854. The central Board of Health was <u>dismantled</u> in 1858.

Snow linked Cholera to Contaminated Water

<u>John Snow</u> showed that there was a connection between <u>contaminated water</u> and <u>cholera</u> in 1853-54. He studied a cholera outbreak in the <u>Broad Street</u> area of London and noticed that the victims all used the <u>same water pump</u>. So he removed the <u>handle</u> from the pump and ended the outbreak.

Snow's work received <u>little attention</u> at first. Most people still believed diseases were spread by <u>miasma</u> ('bad air').

Public Health

These activities will help you understand the impact poor public health had on Britain in the 19th century.

Knowledge and Understanding

1) Copy and complete the mind map below, explaining how each factor affected public health in the 19th century.

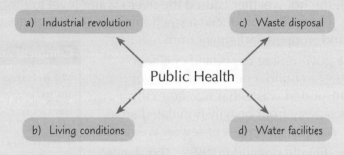

a) Industrial revolution

c) Waste disposal

Public Health

b) Living conditions

d) Water facilities

2) Explain what cholera is and the effect it had on people in Britain during the 19th century.

3) Summarise the findings of Chadwick's 1842 report.

4) Give two reasons why the 1848 Public Health Act had little impact on public health.

5) Explain why John Snow's work was important for public health.

Source Analysis

The source on the right is a cartoon that was published in a British magazine in 1866.

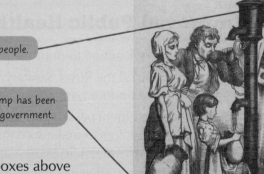

a) Death is pumping water for people.

b) The caption claims that the pump has been provided for the poor by the local government.

1) Explain what each detail in the blue boxes above suggests about public health in the 19th century.

2) Explain how the date of this source affects its usefulness for an investigation into public health in the 19th century.

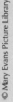

DEATH'S DISPENSARY.
OPEN TO THE POOR, GRATIS, BY PERMISSION OF THE PARISH.

© Mary Evans Picture Library

If anyone knows the cause of cholera, John Snows...

EXAM TIP

When you're explaining the significance of a development, you can show the examiner how well you understand it by writing about both its short-term and long-term consequences.

A Revolution in Medicine

Public Health

Despite the work of Chadwick and Snow, public health didn't improve — cholera returned to Britain in 1865. But then, thanks to several factors, things began to change and the government took action.

The 'Great Stink' struck London in 1858

1) As in other towns, a lot of waste in London drained into water sources, including the River Thames.

2) In the summer of 1858, the hot weather caused the river's water level to drop and bacteria to grow in the waste. This produced a smell that was so bad it affected large parts of London and stopped Parliament from meeting.

3) To reduce the stink, the government appointed engineer Joseph Bazalgette in 1859 to build a new London sewer system. The sewers transported waste that was normally dumped into the Thames away from heavily populated areas to the Thames Estuary. About 1300 miles of sewers were built.

4) The sewer system was officially opened in 1865. Bazalgette's design became the blueprint for most cities in Western Europe.

> **Comment and Analysis**
>
> When Bazalgette started work on his sewers, people still didn't understand how diseases spread. They were trying to get rid of the bad smells coming from the Thames. The fact they stopped cholera in London by cleaning the drinking water was unintended.

Public Opinion began to Change

For most of the 19th century, people believed in a laissez-faire style of government — they thought the government shouldn't intervene in public health. But then things began to change.

1) Evidence from Chadwick and Snow (see p.44), and Pasteur's Germ Theory (see p.36), showed that cleaning towns could stop the spread of disease.

2) In 1867, the Second Reform Act was passed giving nearly 1 million more men the vote, most of whom were industrial workers.

3) Several reformers helped change attitudes towards health. William Farr was a statistician who recorded causes of death. He used his statistics to press for reforms in areas where death rates were high.

> Now they had the vote, workers could put pressure on the government to listen to concerns about health. For the first time, politicians had to address workers' concerns in order to stay in power.

The 1875 Act improved Public Health

In the 1870s the government finally took action to improve public health.

1) In 1871-72, the government followed the Royal Sanitary Commission's proposal to form the Local Government Board and divide Britain into 'sanitary areas' administered by officers for public health.

2) In 1875, Benjamin Disraeli's government passed another Public Health Act. It forced councils to appoint health inspectors and sanitary inspectors to make sure that laws on things like water supplies and hygiene were followed. It also made councils maintain sewerage systems and keep their towns' streets clean.

3) The 1875 Public Health Act was more effective than the one passed in 1848 because it was compulsory.

4) Disraeli also brought in the Artisans' Dwellings Act in 1875. This let local councils buy slums with poor living conditions and rebuild them in a way that fit new government-backed housing standards.

> Few councillors used the Artisans' Dwellings Act. An exception was Joseph Chamberlain, who became Mayor of Birmingham in 1873. Chamberlain persuaded the city authorities to buy the local gas and water companies to make sure people had good supplies of both. In 1875, he cleared an area of the city's slums and built a new street in their place. He also improved some of the slum housing.

> **Comment and Analysis**
>
> There were several changes to public health during the industrial revolution, and the 1875 Public Health Act was the biggest. The work of the government and individuals like Chadwick, Snow and Farr were key to these changes. Technology (like Bazalgette's sewers), the 1867 Reform Act and the cholera epidemics were other factors that prompted improvement.

A Revolution in Medicine

Public Health

The government began to get more involved in trying to improve sanitation in towns and cities. Try these activities to check you understand what the government did to help make Britain a cleaner place.

Knowledge and Understanding

1) In your own words, explain what the 'Great Stink' was.

2) Copy and complete the mind map below, giving reasons why attitudes towards the government's involvement in public health began to change in the 19th century.

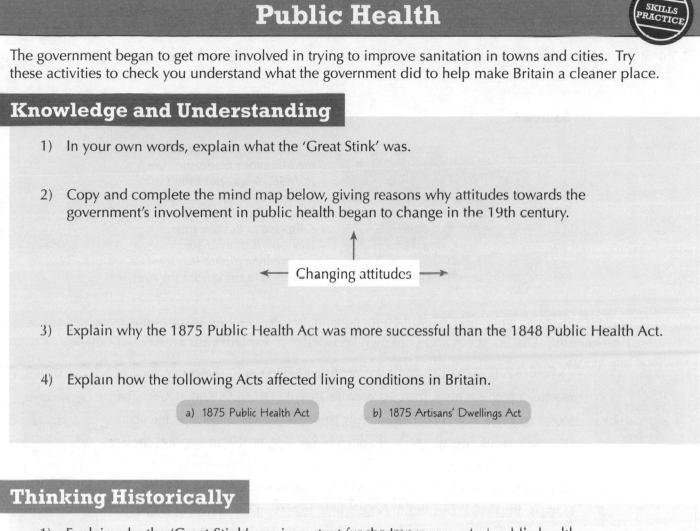

Changing attitudes

3) Explain why the 1875 Public Health Act was more successful than the 1848 Public Health Act.

4) Explain how the following Acts affected living conditions in Britain.

a) 1875 Public Health Act   b) 1875 Artisans' Dwellings Act

Thinking Historically

1) Explain why the 'Great Stink' was important for the improvement of public health.

2) Which of the following factors do you think was the most important in ending cholera outbreaks in London? Explain your answer.

chance   individuals   the government

You should refer to all three factors in your answer. Use pages 44 and 46 to help you.

3) Copy and complete the table below, adding evidence for and against the following statement: 'The work of individuals has been the most important factor in improving public health between c.1800 and c.1900'. You can use information from throughout this section.

For	Against

EXAM TIP

Turns out laissez-faire had made things less fair...

Make sure that you're comfortable talking about a range of factors. These factors include individuals, the government, religion, science and technology, war, communication and chance.

A Revolution in Medicine

Worked Exam-Style Question

Look at this sample answer and the comments to help you tackle the source-based exam question.

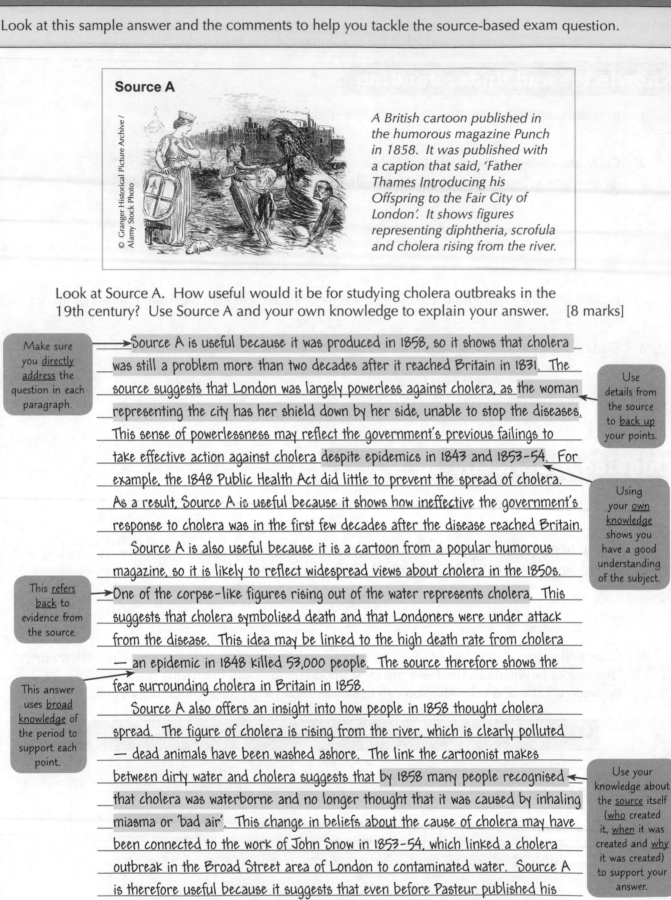

Source A

© Granger Historical Picture Archive / Alamy Stock Photo

A British cartoon published in the humorous magazine Punch in 1858. It was published with a caption that said, 'Father Thames Introducing his Offspring to the Fair City of London'. It shows figures representing diphtheria, scrofula and cholera rising from the river.

Look at Source A. How useful would it be for studying cholera outbreaks in the 19th century? Use Source A and your own knowledge to explain your answer. **[8 marks]**

> Make sure you <u>directly address</u> the question in each paragraph.

> Use details from the source to <u>back up</u> your points.

> Using your <u>own knowledge</u> shows you have a good understanding of the subject.

> This <u>refers back</u> to evidence from the source.

> This answer uses <u>broad knowledge</u> of the period to support each point.

> Use your knowledge about the <u>source</u> itself (<u>who</u> created it, <u>when</u> it was created and <u>why</u> it was created) to support your answer.

Source A is useful because it was produced in 1858, so it shows that cholera was still a problem more than two decades after it reached Britain in 1831. The source suggests that London was largely powerless against cholera, as the woman representing the city has her shield down by her side, unable to stop the diseases. This sense of powerlessness may reflect the government's previous failings to take effective action against cholera despite epidemics in 1843 and 1853-54. For example, the 1848 Public Health Act did little to prevent the spread of cholera. As a result, Source A is useful because it shows how ineffective the government's response to cholera was in the first few decades after the disease reached Britain.

Source A is also useful because it is a cartoon from a popular humorous magazine, so it is likely to reflect widespread views about cholera in the 1850s. One of the corpse-like figures rising out of the water represents cholera. This suggests that cholera symbolised death and that Londoners were under attack from the disease. This idea may be linked to the high death rate from cholera — an epidemic in 1848 killed 53,000 people. The source therefore shows the fear surrounding cholera in Britain in 1858.

Source A also offers an insight into how people in 1858 thought cholera spread. The figure of cholera is rising from the river, which is clearly polluted — dead animals have been washed ashore. The link the cartoonist makes between dirty water and cholera suggests that by 1858 many people recognised that cholera was waterborne and no longer thought that it was caused by inhaling miasma or 'bad air'. This change in beliefs about the cause of cholera may have been connected to the work of John Snow in 1853-54, which linked a cholera outbreak in the Broad Street area of London to contaminated water. Source A is therefore useful because it suggests that even before Pasteur published his Germ Theory in 1861, miasma theory was being challenged, at least in relation to certain diseases, such as cholera.

Exam-Style Questions

Give these questions a go to make sure you understand how medicine changed in the 19th century.

Source A

An extract from 'An Inquiry into the Sanitary Condition of the Labouring Population of Great Britain,' by Edwin Chadwick, which was presented to Parliament in 1842. This report was based on work done by a team of commissioners led by Chadwick, who travelled the country to find out what life was like for poor people.

> The various forms of epidemic... and other disease... chiefly amongst the labouring classes [are caused] by atmospheric impurities produced by decomposing animal and vegetable substances, by damp and filth, and close and overcrowded dwellings...
>
> As to the means by which sanitary conditions of the labouring classes may be improved: — The primary and most important measures, and at the same time the most practicable... are drainage, the removal of all refuse* of habitations**, streets, and roads, and the improvement of the supplies of water.

*waste   **homes

Exam-Style Questions

1) Look at Source A. How useful would it be for studying public health in 19th-century Britain? Use Source A and your own knowledge to explain your answer. [8 marks]

2) Explain why the work of Louis Pasteur was important for the development of medicine. [8 marks]

3) Explain the similarities between public health during the Middle Ages and during the industrial revolution. [8 marks]

4) Has the role of individuals been the most important factor in the development of surgery since the Middle Ages? Explain your answer.

   For the 16-mark question in the exam, 4 extra marks will be available for spelling, punctuation, grammar and using specialist terminology.

   Your answer should discuss the role of individuals and other factors. Make sure you include examples from across the period c.1000 to the present day. [16 marks]

The Impact of the First World War

The First World War (1914-1918) caused devastation in Europe. But the soldiers' injuries gave surgeons opportunities to find new techniques for diagnosis and for carrying out more complex operations.

The First World War made X-rays more Reliable and Mobile

Wilhelm Röntgen discovered X-rays in 1895. X-rays pass easily through soft flesh, but less well through bone. X-ray images could therefore be produced by directing X-rays at a body part in front of a photographic plate.

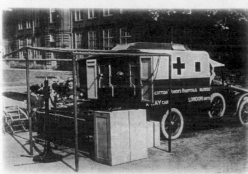

A photograph from 1915, showing a First World War hospital car equipped with mobile X-ray equipment.

1) X-rays were used from the start of the First World War to find broken bones, but the equipment included glass tubes that were unreliable and often stopped working. Also, it was often located in hospitals miles away from the battlefields.

2) The American scientist William Coolidge had invented a more reliable X-ray tube in 1913. The 'Coolidge tube' became widely used by the end of the war, and is still used today.

3) In 1914, the Polish scientist Marie Curie developed mobile X-ray units (ambulances equipped with X-ray machines) which allowed doctors to transport X-ray equipment.

> The war also increased the number of radiologists — people who know how to operate X-ray equipment. Curie and French scientist Antoine Béclère set up training schools to teach doctors how to use X-ray equipment.

The problem of Blood Loss was overcome as a result of the war

The idea of blood transfusions was known from the 17th century, but they were rarely successful because the blood of the recipient often clotted. Blood also clotted if it was stored outside the body.

1) In 1900, Karl Landsteiner discovered blood groups. Certain blood groups couldn't be mixed together as the blood would clot, blocking the blood vessels. Landsteiner's discovery meant doctors could perform more successful blood transfusions, as long as the donor's blood group was the same as the patient's.

2) During World War I the seriousness of wounds from gunshots and explosive shells meant that many soldiers died of blood loss. This made being able to store blood very important.

3) In 1914, doctors found that sodium citrate stopped blood clotting so it could be stored. In 1917, this discovery allowed the first ever blood depot to be set up at the Battle of Cambrai.

4) In 1946, the British National Blood Transfusion Service was established.

> Patients always suffer some blood loss during surgery. If a lot of blood is lost, this can be fatal. Blood transfusions helped to prevent this cause of death by enabling surgeons to replace any blood lost during surgery.

War sped up the development of Plastic Surgery

1) Doctors in France and Germany had been working on skin graft techniques since before the First World War. Their work helped pave the way for Harold Gillies, who set up a plastic surgery unit for the British Army during the war.

2) Gillies was interested in reconstructing facial injuries so that patients could have a normal appearance. He developed the use of pedicle tubes, and kept detailed records of his achievements.

> A pedicle tube is a skin graft technique where skin is partially cut from a healthy part of a patient's body, grown and then attached to the damaged area of the patient to cover any scarring.

3) Gillies' work was continued during the Second World War by his assistant, Archibald McIndoe. A lot of McIndoe's patients were pilots who had been trapped inside burning aircraft.

The Impact of the First World War

Many important developments linked to X-rays, blood transfusions and plastic surgery happened as a result of the First World War. Make sure you know these developments by doing the activities below.

Knowledge and Understanding

1) Copy and complete the mind map below, describing the role that each individual played in the development of X-rays.

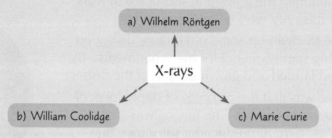

a) Wilhelm Röntgen

X-rays

b) William Coolidge

c) Marie Curie

2) Give two reasons why blood transfusions were rarely successful before the 20th century.

3) Explain why each of the following developments helped to make blood transfusions more successful.

a) Karl Landsteiner's discovery of blood groups

b) The use of sodium citrate

4) Why did the development of blood transfusions make surgery safer?

5) How did Harold Gillies improve plastic surgery?

Thinking Historically

1) Copy and complete the table below, explaining why the First World War was important for the development of each medical technique.

Medical technique	Importance of the First World War
a) **X-rays**	
b) **Blood transfusions**	
c) **Plastic surgery**	

2) Do you think war or individuals played a more important role in the development of the medical techniques above? Explain your answer, referring to both factors.

EXAM TIP

Doctors search for broken bones — X-ray marks the spot...

Think about what people would have known at the time. The link between blood groups and blood transfusions is known by doctors today, but it wasn't known to people before 1900.

Penicillin

In the 1800s, Pasteur discovered that <u>bacteria</u> cause disease. But it wasn't until the 1900s that doctors were able to <u>treat</u> bacterial diseases. This was partly due to the discovery of <u>penicillin</u>, the first <u>antibiotic</u>.

Fleming discovered Penicillin — the first Antibiotic

1) <u>Alexander Fleming</u> saw many soldiers die of septic wounds caused by <u>staphylococcal</u> bacteria when he was working in an army hospital during the <u>First World War</u>.

2) Searching for a cure he identified the <u>antiseptic</u> substance in tears, <u>lysozyme</u>, in 1922 — but this only worked on <u>some</u> germs.

3) One day in 1928 he came to clean up some old <u>culture dishes</u> on which he had been growing <u>staphylococci</u> for his experiments. By chance, a <u>fungal spore</u> had landed and grown on one of the dishes.

4) What caught Fleming's eye was that the <u>colonies</u> of staphylococci around the <u>mould</u> had stopped growing. The <u>fungus</u> was identified as <u>Penicillium notatum</u>. It produced a substance that <u>killed</u> bacteria. This substance was given the name <u>penicillin</u>.

5) Fleming <u>published</u> his findings in articles between 1929 and 1931. However, <u>nobody</u> was willing to <u>fund</u> further research, so he was <u>unable</u> to take his work further. The industrial production of penicillin still needed to be developed.

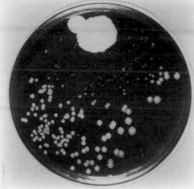

© Mary Evans Picture Library

The original plate on which Fleming first observed the growth of Penicillium notatum.

Florey and Chain found a way to Purify Penicillin

1) Since it is a natural product, penicillin needs to be <u>purified</u>. A breakthrough was made by <u>Howard Florey's</u> team in Oxford between 1938 and 1940. <u>Ernst Chain</u>, a member of the team, devised the <u>freeze-drying</u> technique which was an important part of the purification process.

2) At first Florey and Chain <u>didn't</u> have the <u>resources</u> to produce penicillin in large amounts. They made penicillin for their first <u>clinical trial</u> by growing <u>Penicillium notatum</u> in every container they could find in their lab. Their patient began to recover, only to die when the penicillin <u>ran out</u>.

Florey took penicillin to America for Mass Production

Florey knew that <u>penicillin</u> could be vital in treating the <u>wounds</u> of soldiers fighting in World War II. British <u>chemical firms</u> were too busy making <u>explosives</u> to start mass production — so he went to <u>America</u>.

1) American firms were also not keen to help — until America <u>joined the war</u> in 1941. In December 1941, the US government began to give out <u>grants</u> to businesses that <u>manufactured</u> penicillin.

2) By 1943, British businesses had also started <u>mass-producing</u> penicillin. Mass production was sufficient for the needs of the <u>military medics</u> by 1944.

3) After the war, the <u>cost</u> of penicillin fell, making it more accessible for <u>general use</u>.

4) Fleming, Florey and Chain were awarded the <u>Nobel Prize</u> in 1945.

> Today, penicillin is used to treat a <u>range</u> of <u>bacterial</u> infections, including chest infections and skin infections. Other <u>antibiotics</u> were discovered after 1945, including treatments for lung infections, acne and bacterial meningitis.

Comment and Analysis

While <u>individuals</u> (like Florey, Chain and Fleming) were important in making the discovery of penicillin, it was large institutions like <u>governments</u> that funded its mass production.

Penicillin

The discovery and mass production of penicillin were important developments in medicine — but they didn't happen overnight. Try these activities to make sure you know what happened when.

Knowledge and Understanding

1) What is penicillin and why is it important?

2) Explain how Fleming discovered penicillin. Use the key words from the boxes below.

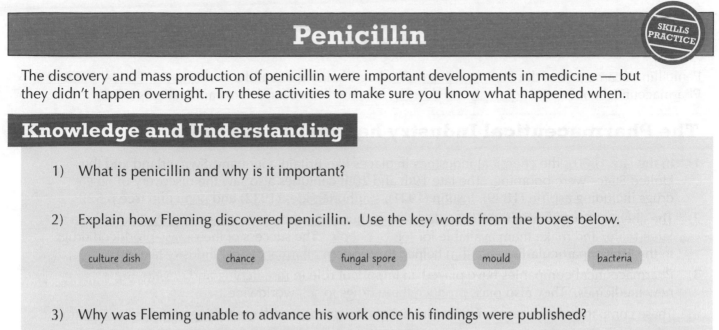

culture dish   chance   fungal spore   mould   bacteria

3) Why was Fleming unable to advance his work once his findings were published?

4) Why was Florey and Chain's first clinical trial of penicillin unsuccessful? Give as much detail as you can.

Thinking Historically

1) Copy and complete the diagram below, explaining the consequence of each event for the development of penicillin. Try to include as much detail as possible.

Fleming sees soldiers die of septic wounds.	a) Consequence:
Chain devises a freeze-drying technique.	b) Consequence:
America joins World War II.	c) Consequence:
The cost of producing penicillin falls.	d) Consequence:

2) Explain how each of the following factors contributed to the success of penicillin.

a) war   b) chance   c) government

3) Which of the factors above do you think was the most important for the success of penicillin? Explain your answer.

EXAM
TIP

Penicillin isn't just mould news — it's still used today...

You should write out a quick plan for the longer question at the end of the paper. This will help you to cover all of the key points and make sure your argument is coherent and well structured.

Modern Treatments

Penicillin became one of the first <u>mass-produced</u> drugs, helping to build a new <u>pharmaceutical industry</u>. Pharmaceutical companies <u>research</u> and <u>develop</u> new medicines for doctors and patients to use.

The Pharmaceutical Industry has really taken off

1) In the <u>late 1800s</u>, the <u>chemical industries</u> in places like Britain, Germany, Switzerland and the United States were booming. The late 19th and 20th centuries also saw the discovery of new drugs including <u>aspirin</u> (1899), <u>insulin</u> (1921), <u>sulphonamides</u> (1932) and <u>penicillin</u> (see p.52).

2) The chemical companies were best placed to <u>manufacture</u> these new <u>drugs and medicines</u> on a <u>large scale</u>, and make them available for <u>lots of people</u>. The success of their <u>mass-produced</u> drugs in the 1940s (particularly <u>penicillin</u>) helped the modern <u>pharmaceutical industry</u> take off.

3) Pharmaceutical companies have played an important role in <u>researching</u> and <u>developing</u> new medicines. They also <u>mass produce</u> these drugs to <u>sell</u> worldwide.

4) These companies have been important in curing <u>new diseases</u> and researching <u>new forms of treatment</u>:

- <u>Chemotherapy</u> is the treatment of cancer using <u>drugs</u>. It began to be developed during <u>World War II</u>, and pharmaceutical companies have been producing cancer drugs since the 1960s.
- In <u>1981</u>, doctors identified a <u>new</u> illness, <u>AIDS</u>, which is caused by the <u>HIV</u> virus. In 1987, pharmaceutical companies began mass producing a drug called <u>AZT</u>, the first approved drug to <u>treat HIV</u>. They have since been involved in developing <u>more effective</u> treatments for HIV.
- In <u>2002</u>, there was an outbreak of a <u>new virus</u> called <u>SARS</u> in China. The virus <u>quickly spread</u> to many different countries. SARS can cause severe <u>breathing difficulties</u> that are sometimes <u>fatal</u>. To date there is <u>no cure</u> for SARS, but companies produce treatments that reduce the symptoms.

The pharmaceutical industry has faced several Problems

1) Drugs have to go through a series of <u>clinical tests</u> before they are given to patients. This is to make sure that they <u>work properly</u> and don't cause any damaging <u>side-effects</u>.

- In the 1950s, the drug <u>thalidomide</u> was released without thorough testing. It was originally used as a <u>sleeping pill</u>, but it soon became popular among pregnant women as a treatment for <u>morning sickness</u>. Tragically, thalidomide affected the women's <u>unborn babies</u>, causing thousands of children to be born with <u>under-developed limbs</u> and other issues.
- The <u>thalidomide tragedy</u> forced pharmaceutical companies to test drugs more thoroughly. The <u>government</u> responded to the tragedy in 1963 by setting up a <u>Committee on Safety of Drugs</u> to make sure all new drugs were <u>safe</u> before being given to patients.

2) Pharmaceutical companies have <u>high costs</u> for research and development of new medicines. <u>Rare diseases</u> sometimes go <u>unresearched</u> because companies tend to focus on treatments for <u>common diseases</u> that will make <u>a lot of money</u>.

3) <u>Antibiotic resistance</u> is when a type of bacteria adapts so it <u>isn't affected</u> by antibiotics anymore. This resistance develops when doctors and patients <u>overuse</u> antibiotics — the more antibiotics are used, the more likely it is that bacteria will become resistant to them.

- <u>Antibiotic resistance</u> stops antibiotics from working properly, making it more difficult to treat some diseases. This has <u>increased</u> the <u>levels of disease</u> and the time taken for patients to recover.
- Around <u>25,000 people</u> in the European Union die every year as a result of infections caused by antibiotic-resistant bacteria.

Modern Treatments

Make sure you know the impact the pharmaceutical industry has had on medicine with these activities.

Knowledge and Understanding

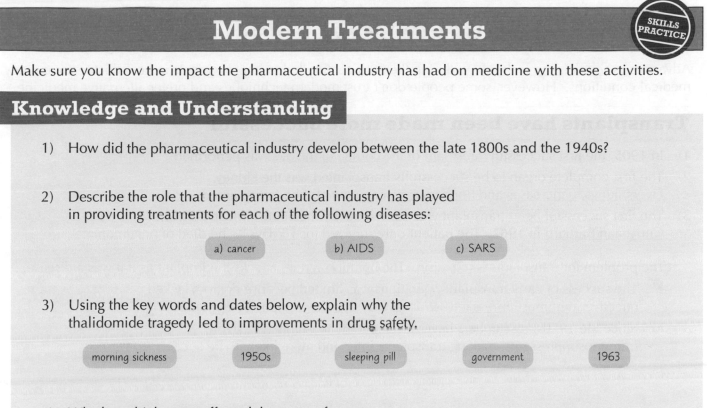

1) How did the pharmaceutical industry develop between the late 1800s and the 1940s?

2) Describe the role that the pharmaceutical industry has played
    in providing treatments for each of the following diseases:

    a) cancer   b) AIDS   c) SARS

3) Using the key words and dates below, explain why the
    thalidomide tragedy led to improvements in drug safety.

    morning sickness   1950s   sleeping pill   government   1963

4) Why have high costs affected the types of treatments
    pharmaceutical companies research and develop?

Source Analysis

The source below is from a newspaper article that was published in 2018 when Public
Health England (a government organisation that aims to improve people's health) launched
its 'Keep Antibiotics Working' campaign. In this extract, Professor Paul Cosford, who is the
medical director of Public Health England, is discussing the overuse of antibiotics.

> "It is concerning that, in the not-too distant future, we may see more cancer patients,
> mothers who've had caesareans* and patients who've had other surgery facing life-threatening
> situations if antibiotics fail to ward off infections.
>
> "We need to preserve antibiotics for when we really need them and we are calling on the
> public to join us in tackling antibiotic resistance by listening to your GP, pharmacist or nurse's
> advice and only taking antibiotics when necessary. Taking antibiotics just in case may seem like
> a harmless act but it can have grave consequences for you and your family's health in future."

*a type of surgery used to deliver babies

1) Imagine you are using this source for an investigation into antibiotic resistance.
    Explain how each feature of the source below affects its usefulness for your investigation.

    a) Author   b) Content   c) Purpose

Farmaceutical companies work on animal treatments...

*Just because a concept or topic is modern, it doesn't mean you should assume the examiner
knows what you're talking about. You still need to back up your points with solid examples.*

Modern Treatments

Advances in science and technology during the 20th century led to improvements in how doctors treat many medical conditions. However, some people don't trust modern techniques and prefer alternative medicine.

Transplants have been made more Successful

1) In 1905, the first successful transplant of the cornea of the eye was performed.

2) The first complete organ to be successfully transplanted was the kidney.
   Livers, lungs, pancreases and bone marrow can now also be transplanted.

3) The first successful heart transplant was carried out by the South African surgeon
   Christiaan Barnard in 1967. The patient only survived for 18 days — he died of pneumonia.

   The problem for transplants is rejection. The immune system attacks the implant as if it was a disease.
   - The success of early transplant operations was limited because doctors lacked
     effective immunosuppressants   drugs that stop the immune system attacking.
   - Since the 1970s, researchers have developed increasingly effective
     immunosuppressants, making transplants safer and more likely to be successful.

Technology has improved modern surgery

1) Advances in science and technology have led to improvements in the treatment of diseases like cancer.
   The discovery of radiation in 1896-1898 by Antoine Henri Becquerel, Marie Curie and Pierre Curie
   led to the creation of radiation therapy. Radiation therapy is the use of radiation to kill cancer cells.

2) The development of lasers since the 1950s led to their widespread use in medicine in the 1980s. Laser
   surgery is used to correct vision problems, and lasers are also used in cancer treatment and dentistry.

3) Advances in video technology led to the development of keyhole surgery in the 1980s.

   - A type of camera called an endoscope is put through a small cut, letting the surgeon see inside
     the body. Other surgical instruments are then introduced through even smaller cuts in the skin.
   - Keyhole surgery is useful for investigating the causes of pain or infertility. It's also used for
     vasectomies, removing cysts or the appendix, mending hernias and other minor operations.
   - Keyhole surgery leaves patients with smaller scars and allows
     them to recover more quickly, with less risk of infection.

Some people use Alternative Treatments

1) Mistrust of modern medicine and technology means some people use alternative therapies instead.
   - Acupuncture is the method of putting needles in specific points of the patient's skin to relieve pain.
   - Homeopathy is treatment using extremely weak solutions of natural substances.

2) Unlike mainstream treatments, alternative therapies aren't based on evidence gathered from
   scientific research. As a result, there is little scientific evidence that alternative treatments
   work effectively, and some doctors believe that they might do more harm than good.

3) However, some doctors are now working with alternative therapists to see if using a
   mix of alternative and mainstream medicine might result in benefits to the patient.

Modern Treatments

Here are some more activities on modern medical treatments. These ones will help you get to grips with developments in surgery, medical technology and alternative treatments during the 20th and 21st centuries.

Knowledge and Understanding

1) Explain the significance of immunosuppressants in modern surgery.

2) Describe how the following advances in technology have affected medical treatments:

a) Radiation   b) Lasers

3) Using the key words below, explain how advances in video technology have affected surgery.

recovery   endoscope   keyhole   scars   minor operations   infection

4) Describe two alternative therapies.

5) How are alternative treatments different from mainstream treatments?

Thinking Historically

1) Copy and complete the table below, describing changes to surgery during 19th century (see pages 40 and 42) and changes during the 20th century (see pages 50 and 56).

Surgery in the 19th century	Surgery in the 20th century

2) Do you think the most important changes to surgery took place during the 19th century or the 20th century? Explain your answer, using the table above to help you.

3) Copy and complete these mind maps, comparing the role of barber-surgeons (see page 14) and modern surgeons.

Think about their knowledge and training, their contribution to medical developments and social attitudes to surgeons.

← barber-surgeons →   ← modern surgeons →

EXAM TIP

All you need to do is transplant these facts into your brain...

To hit the top marks on the last question of the paper, you need to go beyond the factor mentioned in the question. You can use it as a starting point, but write about other factors too.

The Liberal Social Reforms

In the 19th century, people believed government should have little involvement in public health. This all began to change after 1900, when the Liberal social reforms were introduced to deal with poverty.

Booth and Rowntree showed the effects of Poverty

1) Slums and other poor, overcrowded housing were all still common in industrial towns in 1900. The poor worked long hours for low wages. Many people couldn't afford doctors or medicine — they could barely provide their children with three decent meals a day.

> There was no unemployment benefit, or pensions for the elderly. Workhouses were the only help — they provided basic food and lodging in exchange for working long hours in brutal conditions.

2) Two reports showed how widespread poverty was:

Booth's Report

Charles Booth's 1889 'Life and Labour of the People in London' showed that 30% of Londoners were living in severe poverty, and that it was sometimes impossible for people to find work, however hard they tried. He showed that some wages were so low they weren't enough to support a family.

Rowntree's Report

Seebohm Rowntree had a factory in York. He didn't believe the problem was as bad there as in London — so he did a survey of living conditions. His report, 'Poverty, a Study of Town Life' (published 1901), showed that 28% of people in York couldn't afford basic food and housing.

3) The lack of access to good healthcare meant that most people's health was pretty poor. When the Boer War broke out in 1899, army officers found that 40% of volunteers were physically unfit for military service — mostly due to poverty-related illnesses linked to poor diet and living conditions.

4) The government realised that it needed to improve basic healthcare in order to have an efficient army.

The Liberal Reforms improved health by tackling Poverty

Booth, Rowntree and the Boer War showed that there was a link between poverty and ill health. The newly-elected Liberal government and its Chancellor, David Lloyd George, realised it had to take action.

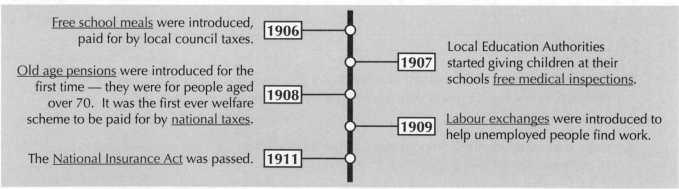

Free school meals were introduced, paid for by local council taxes. **1906**

1907 Local Education Authorities started giving children at their schools free medical inspections.

Old age pensions were introduced for the first time — they were for people aged over 70. It was the first ever welfare scheme to be paid for by national taxes. **1908**

1909 Labour exchanges were introduced to help unemployed people find work.

The National Insurance Act was passed. **1911**

The National Insurance Act introduced health insurance for workers — the worker, their employer and the government all contributed to a central fund that the workers could use for sick pay or to pay for a doctor.

Comment and Analysis

The Liberal reforms were the first real effort by the national government to improve people's living conditions as a way of improving their health. The reforms were a result of changing attitudes towards the role of government, and changed people's attitudes further.

The Liberal Social Reforms

Check that you know all about the Liberal reforms and the events that led to them with these activities.

Knowledge and Understanding

1) What did each of the following reports reveal about poverty in Britain?

    a) 'Life and Labour of the People in London' by Charles Booth

    b) 'Poverty, a Study of Town Life' by Seebohm Rowntree

2) Why do you think Booth and Rowntree's reports encouraged the government to become more involved in public health?

3) Explain why the Boer War was important for public health in Britain.

4) Describe how the Liberal reforms affected each of the following groups:

    a) Children   b) Elderly people   c) Unemployed people   d) Workers

Source Analysis

The source below is a leaflet that was published by the Liberal government in 1911.
It shows David Lloyd George sitting with an ill worker. The caption reads 'Mr. Lloyd George's National Health Insurance Bill provides for the insurance of the Worker in case of Sickness'.

1) Why do you think the government chose to use an image of Lloyd George sitting with an ill worker in this leaflet?

2) What impression does the source create of the Liberal reforms? Support your answer with details from the source.

3) Why do you think the Liberal government wanted to create this impression of the Liberal reforms? Use your own knowledge to explain your answer.

4) How useful do you think this source would be for an investigation into attitudes towards the Liberal reforms? Explain your answer.

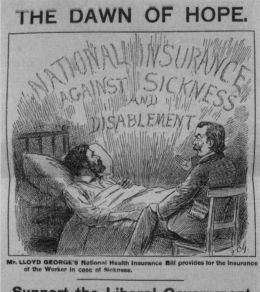

THE DAWN OF HOPE.

NATIONAL INSURANCE AGAINST SICKNESS AND DISABLEMENT

Mr. LLOYD GEORGE'S National Health Insurance Bill provides for the insurance of the Worker in case of Sickness.

Support the Liberal Government
in their policy of
SOCIAL REFORM.

Poverty, a Study of Town Life — not a holiday read...

In the exam, you only have a limited amount of time to answer each question. If you're spending too long on one question, finish your point then move on to the next question.

Public Health and the World Wars

After World War II, housing standards began to improve. The Beveridge Report argued that the state should provide support to people, resulting in the creation of the welfare state and the NHS.

The World Wars created Pressure for Social Change

The First World War (1914-1918) and the Second World War (1939-1945) broke down social distinctions and brought people together whose lives had been very separate.

1) Raising mass armies made government and military officials more aware of the health problems of the poor, because so many recruits were in poor health. Powerful people were more concerned with solving these health problems when at war, because of the need for a strong army to defend the country.

2) The evacuation of children during the Second World War increased awareness in richer rural communities of how disadvantaged many people were in other parts of the country.

3) After the Second World War, people looked for improvements in society. Such feelings led to the 1945 victory for the Labour Party, which promised healthcare for everyone and full employment.

Housing and Health Improved after the Second World War

1) Towards the end of the First World War, Prime Minister David Lloyd George promised to tackle poor-quality housing by building 'homes fit for heroes' to tackle bad housing. Some new council houses were built in the 1920s and 1930s, but many of them were too expensive for the poorest families, who still lived in slums.

2) During the Second World War, destruction from bombing and a lack of construction led to severe housing shortages, making the situation worse.

3) After the war, the Labour government built 800,000 homes between 1945-51. In 1946, it passed the New Towns Act — this created completely new towns near major cities. Governments in the 1950s and 1960s demolished over 900,000 old, cramped slums — around 2 million inhabitants were rehoused.

4) In 1961, a report called 'Homes for Today and Tomorrow' gave specific standards for new housing, including adequate heating, a flushing toilet and enough space inside and outside. This was the final step in tackling the issues of overcrowding, poor nutrition and poor waste disposal that had caused major public health problems.

The Beveridge Report led to the Welfare State

1) In 1942, during the Second World War, economist and social reformer William Beveridge published his famous report. The Beveridge Report became a bestseller — it was widely read and hugely popular.

> In his report, Beveridge called for the state provision of social security 'from the cradle to the grave.' Beveridge argued that all people should have the right to be free from want, disease, ignorance, squalor and idleness. He called these the five 'giants.'

2) Beveridge said that the government had a duty to care for all its citizens, not just the poor or unemployed. To achieve this, Beveridge suggested the creation of a welfare state — a system of grants and services available to all British citizens.

3) The 1945 Labour government was elected with the promise to implement Beveridge's proposals. One of their first acts was to pass a new National Insurance Act in 1946 to support anyone who couldn't work, whether as a result of sickness, pregnancy, unemployment or old age.

Comment and Analysis

The Labour Party's National Insurance Act went further than the one introduced by the Liberal government (see p.58) — anyone could apply for Labour's National Insurance without having to take a test to see if they were eligible.

Public Health and the World Wars

The World Wars led to improvements to public health. Complete the activities on this page to check you know the changes that happened and the impact these changes had on the health of the British public.

Knowledge and Understanding

1) How successfully did the government tackle the problem of poor-quality housing after the First World War? Explain your answer.

2) For each of the dates below, describe the development that affected housing. Give as much detail as possible.
   a) 1939-1945
   b) 1945-1951
   c) 1946
   d) 1950s-1960s
   e) 1961

3) Using the key phrases below, explain the recommendations that William Beveridge made in his 1942 report. Give as much detail as you can.

   social security   five 'giants'   welfare state   all citizens

4) What was the National Insurance Act of 1946?

5) How did the 1946 National Insurance Act differ from the one passed by the Liberal government in 1911? Why do you think they were different?

Thinking Historically

1) Copy and complete the table below, explaining the ways the First World War and the Second World War affected living conditions and public health.

First World War	Second World War

Beveridge Report — it's not about your favourite drink...

For the essay question in the exam, you should include examples from across the period c.1000-present. This will show the examiner you have wide knowledge of the question topic.

National Health Service

One of the most important changes in modern British medicine was the creation of the NHS.

The National Health Service was established in 1948

1) In 1948, the Labour government implemented Beveridge's last proposal — a National Health Service.

2) Aneurin Bevan was the Labour Minister for Health who, after a lot of negotiation, introduced the National Health Service (NHS). The government nationalised hospitals and put them under local authority control. Treatment was made free for all patients. There were arguments for and against the NHS:

For the NHS

- During World War Two the government took control of all hospitals, creating the Emergency Medical Service. Its success led many to support the creation of the NHS.
- The NHS would make medical care free so it was accessible to everyone.
- The NHS guaranteed that hospitals would receive government money, rather than having to rely on charities for money.

Against the NHS

- Many Conservatives opposed the NHS as they believed the cost would be huge.
- Doctors saw themselves as independent professionals — they didn't want to be controlled by the government. They also worried that they would lose a lot of income.
- Many doctors threatened to go on strike in protest against the NHS.

The government finally convinced doctors by offering them a payment for each patient and letting them continue treating fee-paying patients.

The NHS was Very Popular

1) Although many Conservatives were opposed to the creation of the NHS, they couldn't abolish it when they came back into power in 1951 — it was too popular.

2) The NHS increased the number of people with access to healthcare — the number of doctors doubled between 1948 and 1973 to keep up with demand.

3) Today, the NHS provides a range of health services, most of which are free and accessible to everyone. They include accident and emergency care, maternity care and major surgery, as well as pharmacies, dentists, mental health services, sexual health services and general practitioners (GPs).

In the long term, the NHS has contributed to a dramatic improvement in people's health and a rise in life expectancy. In 1951, men could expect to live to 66 and women to 72 — by 2011 this had risen to 79 for men and 83 for women.

Today the NHS faces several Challenges

1) The increase in life expectancy means there are many more older people in Britain today than there were in 1948, who are more likely to suffer from long-term conditions like diabetes and heart disease. They need regular medical attention and require a lot of NHS time and resources.

2) Many people's lifestyle choices are putting strain on the NHS. Smoking, obesity and alcohol consumption can all harm people's health and may require expensive treatment — for example, smoking can cause lung cancer and drinking too much alcohol can cause serious liver disease.

3) Many modern treatments, equipment and medicines are very expensive, and the NHS has had to face rising expectations of what it can and should offer.

4) As a result of all these factors, the cost of the NHS is rising rapidly — in 2015/16 the NHS budget was £116 billion overall. In order to stay within its budget, the NHS sometimes has to make difficult choices about which treatments it can and can't provide.

A 2015 poll suggested that around 60% of British people are satisfied with the NHS, showing that it is still relatively popular.

National Health Service

The NHS was a turning point in British healthcare — check you understand what you've read with this page.

Knowledge and Understanding

1) Describe the role of the following individuals in the creation of the NHS:

   a) William Beveridge

   b) Aneurin Bevan

2) Give three reasons why there was opposition to the creation of the NHS.

3) Explain how the Emergency Medical Service contributed to the creation of the NHS.

4) How has the NHS improved public health? Give as much detail as possible.

5) Copy and complete the mind map below,
   listing the challenges that the NHS faces today.

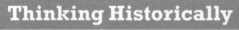

← NHS challenges →

Thinking Historically

1) Copy and complete the mind map below, giving as much detail as you
   can about the government's role in public health during the 19th and
   20th centuries. You can use the information on previous pages to help you.

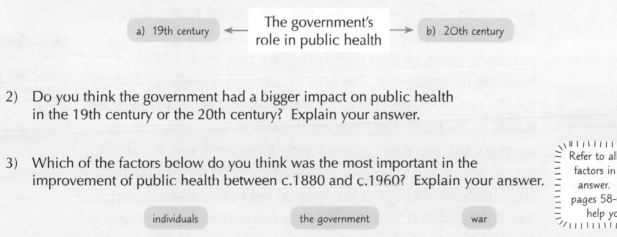

   a) 19th century ← The government's role in public health → b) 20th century

2) Do you think the government had a bigger impact on public health
   in the 19th century or the 20th century? Explain your answer.

3) Which of the factors below do you think was the most important in the
   improvement of public health between c.1880 and c.1960? Explain your answer.

   Refer to all three factors in your answer. Use pages 58-62 to help you.

   individuals   the government   war

EXAM TIP

The NHS has been around for a long while...

*There are many examples of the government's role in healthcare — e.g. the establishment of
the NHS. Don't just give examples in your answer though, explain why they're important.*

Worked Exam-Style Question

This sample answer will help you to write longer answers that focus on the importance of different factors. You need to write a balanced argument that comes to a judgement — look at the comments for help.

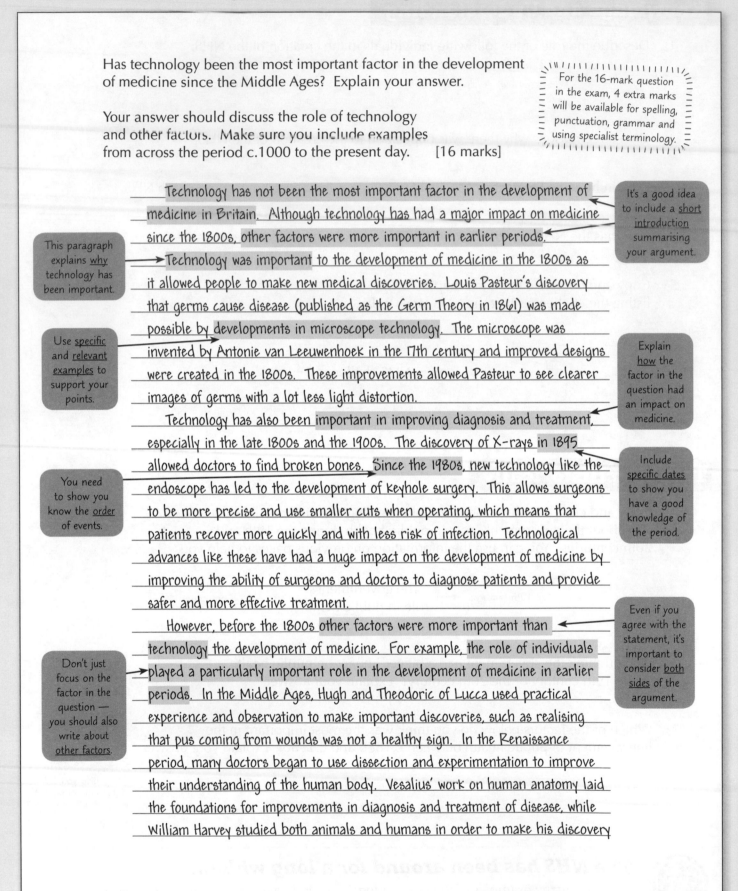

Has technology been the most important factor in the development of medicine since the Middle Ages? Explain your answer.

Your answer should discuss the role of technology and other factors. Make sure you include examples from across the period c.1000 to the present day. [16 marks]

For the 16-mark question in the exam, 4 extra marks will be available for spelling, punctuation, grammar and using specialist terminology.

Technology has not been the most important factor in the development of medicine in Britain. Although technology has had a major impact on medicine since the 1800s, other factors were more important in earlier periods.

Technology was important to the development of medicine in the 1800s as it allowed people to make new medical discoveries. Louis Pasteur's discovery that germs cause disease (published as the Germ Theory in 1861) was made possible by developments in microscope technology. The microscope was invented by Antonie van Leeuwenhoek in the 17th century and improved designs were created in the 1800s. These improvements allowed Pasteur to see clearer images of germs with a lot less light distortion.

Technology has also been important in improving diagnosis and treatment, especially in the late 1800s and the 1900s. The discovery of X-rays in 1895 allowed doctors to find broken bones. Since the 1980s, new technology like the endoscope has led to the development of keyhole surgery. This allows surgeons to be more precise and use smaller cuts when operating, which means that patients recover more quickly and with less risk of infection. Technological advances like these have had a huge impact on the development of medicine by improving the ability of surgeons and doctors to diagnose patients and provide safer and more effective treatment.

However, before the 1800s other factors were more important than technology the development of medicine. For example, the role of individuals played a particularly important role in the development of medicine in earlier periods. In the Middle Ages, Hugh and Theodoric of Lucca used practical experience and observation to make important discoveries, such as realising that pus coming from wounds was not a healthy sign. In the Renaissance period, many doctors began to use dissection and experimentation to improve their understanding of the human body. Vesalius' work on human anatomy laid the foundations for improvements in diagnosis and treatment of disease, while William Harvey studied both animals and humans in order to make his discovery

It's a good idea to include a short introduction summarising your argument.

This paragraph explains why technology has been important.

Use specific and relevant examples to support your points.

Explain how the factor in the question had an impact on medicine.

Include specific dates to show you have a good knowledge of the period.

You need to show you know the order of events.

Even if you agree with the statement, it's important to consider both sides of the argument.

Don't just focus on the factor in the question — you should also write about other factors.

that blood circulates around the body. These individuals helped pave the way for scientists to question old ideas and contribute to new medical developments.

Start a new paragraph every time you introduce a new factor.

Another key factor in the development of medicine was war. For example, many of the surgical techniques invented by Ambroise Paré in the 16th century, such as using ligatures to prevent blood loss after amputation, were devised in response to the injuries he encountered during his time as an army surgeon. War continued to drive medical developments in the 20th century. For example, the First World War led to advances in blood transfusions and plastic surgery as doctors had to find treatments for new injuries.

You should include examples from throughout the thematic study in your answer.

Moreover, while technology has been important since the 1800s, it cannot be considered the most important factor because it has often required economic investment from large institutions like the government in order to have an impact. For example, in the mid-19th century, Bazalgette's new sewer system, which helped to stop cholera in London by cleaning up the city's drinking water, was only built because the government supported the project. Similarly, since the mid-20th century, access to modern medical technology has relied on funding from the National Health Service. Founded in 1948, the NHS provides free access to a range of medical services, including expensive medical equipment. In 2015/16 the NHS budget was £116 billion, showing how much it invests in resources, including technology. This demonstrates that technology has mainly had an impact on the development of medicine when it is supported by the economic resources of large institutions like the government.

Explain how each point you make is relevant to the question.

Use specific facts and figures that are relevant to your argument.

Remember to explain the significance of each factor you write about.

In conclusion, technology has not been the most important factor in the development of medicine in Britain, because before the 1800s other factors, such as war and the work of individuals to advance medical knowledge, were more important. Even though technology has had a major impact on medicine since the 1800s, it is still not the most important factor, because its impact in this period has relied on other factors, especially government funding.

Make sure you give a clear answer to the question in your conclusion.

Summarise your argument in your conclusion.

Exam-Style Questions

Give these exam-style questions a go to test your knowledge of modern medicine. Remember that you'll need to include information about medicine from earlier periods in some of your answers.

Source A

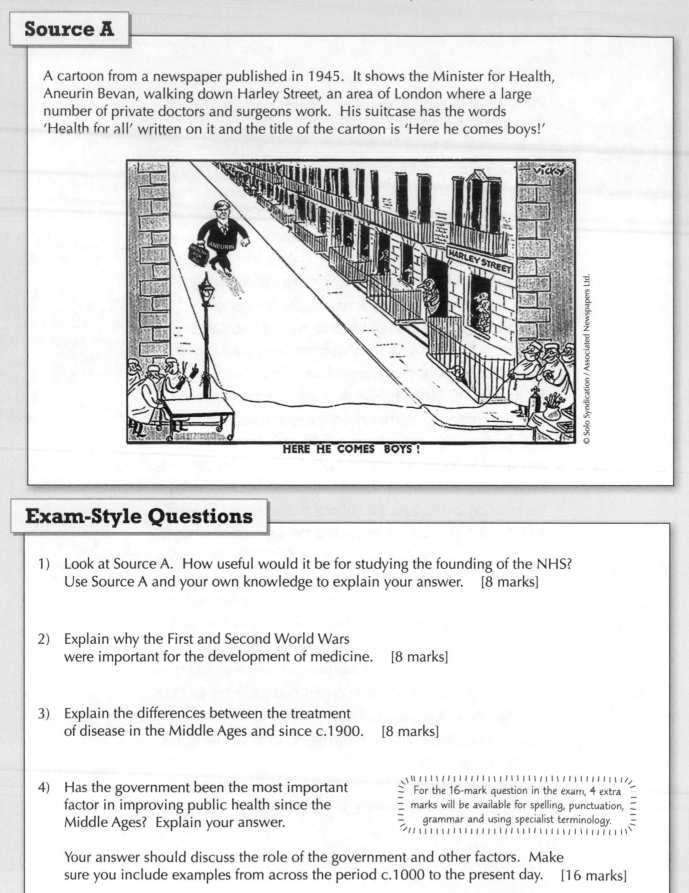

A cartoon from a newspaper published in 1945. It shows the Minister for Health, Aneurin Bevan, walking down Harley Street, an area of London where a large number of private doctors and surgeons work. His suitcase has the words 'Health for all' written on it and the title of the cartoon is 'Here he comes boys!'

HERE HE COMES BOYS !

© Solo Syndication / Associated Newspapers Ltd.

Exam-Style Questions

1) Look at Source A. How useful would it be for studying the founding of the NHS? Use Source A and your own knowledge to explain your answer.   [8 marks]

2) Explain why the First and Second World Wars were important for the development of medicine.   [8 marks]

3) Explain the differences between the treatment of disease in the Middle Ages and since c.1900.   [8 marks]

4) Has the government been the most important factor in improving public health since the Middle Ages? Explain your answer.

> For the 16-mark question in the exam, 4 extra marks will be available for spelling, punctuation, grammar and using specialist terminology.

Your answer should discuss the role of the government and other factors. Make sure you include examples from across the period c.1000 to the present day.   [16 marks]

Answers

Marking the Activities

We've included sample answers for all the activities. When you're marking your work, remember that our answers are just a guide — a lot of the activities ask you to give your own opinion, so there isn't always a 'correct answer'.

Marking the Exam-Style Questions

For each exam-style question, we've covered some key points that your answer could include. Our answers are just examples though — answers very different to ours could also get top marks.

Most exam questions in history are level marked. This means the examiner puts your answer into one of several levels. Then they award marks based on how well your answer matches the description for that level.

To reach a higher level, you'll need to give a 'more sophisticated' answer. Exactly what 'sophisticated' means will depend on the type of question, but, generally speaking, a more sophisticated answer could include more detail, more background knowledge or make a more complex judgement.

Start by choosing which level your answer falls into. If different parts of your answer match different level descriptions, then pick the level description that best matches your answer as a whole. A good way to do this is to start at 'Level 1' and go up to the next level each time your answer meets all the conditions of a level. Next, choose a mark. If your answer completely matches the level description, or parts of it match the level above, give yourself a high mark within the range of the level. If your answer mostly matches the level description, but some parts of it only just match, give yourself a mark in the middle of the range. Award yourself a lower mark within the range if your answer only just meets the conditions for that level or if parts of your answer only match the level below.

Level descriptions:

Source analysis questions:

Level 1 1-2 marks	The answer shows limited understanding of the source and makes a simple statement about its usefulness.
Level 2 3-4 marks	The answer gives a simple analysis of the source's usefulness based on its content and/or provenance. The analysis is supported by basic knowledge and understanding of the topic.
Level 3 5-6 marks	The answer gives a more detailed analysis of the source's usefulness based on its content and/or provenance. The analysis is supported by good knowledge and understanding of the topic.
Level 4 7-8 marks	The answer gives a detailed analysis of the content of the source and its provenance. The analysis is supported by excellent knowledge and understanding of the topic. The answer reaches a well-supported judgement about the usefulness of the source.

Importance questions:

Level 1 1-2 marks	Limited knowledge and understanding of the period is shown. The answer gives a simple explanation of the importance of natural explanations of disease in the Middle Ages.
Level 2 3-4 marks	Some relevant knowledge and understanding of the period is shown. The answer attempts to analyse at least one point about the importance of natural explanations of disease.
Level 3 5-6 marks	A good level of knowledge and understanding is shown. The answer explores two or more points about the importance of natural explanations of disease and analyses them in more detail.
Level 4 7-8 marks	Knowledge and understanding of the period is precise and detailed. The answer explores two or more points about the importance of natural explanations of disease and thoroughly analyses each one. Connections between different points are identified to create a deeper analysis of importance.

Comparison questions:

Level 1 1-2 marks	The answer shows limited knowledge and understanding of the periods. It identifies one or more relevant difference.
Level 2 3-4 marks	The answer shows some knowledge and understanding of the periods. This is used to give a simple explanation of at least one difference.
Level 3 5-6 marks	The answer shows a good level of knowledge and understanding of the periods. This is used to give a more detailed explanation of two or more differences.
Level 4 7-8 marks	The answer shows precise and detailed knowledge and understanding. This is used to analyse two or more differences in detail.

16-mark essay questions:

Level 1 1-4 marks	The answer shows limited relevant knowledge and understanding. One of more factors are explained in a basic way. Ideas aren't organised with an overall argument in mind.
Level 2 5-8 marks	The answer shows some relevant knowledge and understanding. One or more factors are explained in a simple way. Ideas are organised with an overall argument in mind, but the argument isn't well supported by the answer.
Level 3 9-12 marks	The answer shows a good level of relevant knowledge and understanding. It gives a more detailed explanation of the factor in the question and one or more other factors. Most ideas are organised to develop a clear argument that is supported by the answer.
Level 4 13-16 marks	The answer shows an excellent level of relevant knowledge and understanding. It analyses the factor in the question and one or more other factors. All ideas are well organised to develop a clear argument and a well-supported conclusion.

Answers

Medicine Stands Still

Page 7 — Disease and the Supernatural

Knowledge and Understanding

1 a) People prayed and repented for their sins.
   b) Suspected witches were tried and executed.
   c) Exorcisms were performed by members of the Church to remove the evil spirits.
2 Doctors owned an almanac that gave them information about the position of planets and stars. They used this to help them diagnose the causes of a patient's illness by looking at how different star signs affected certain parts of their body.

Thinking Historically

1 a) The Church taught people that disease was a punishment from God for sinful behaviour. This encouraged people to pray and repent to try to cure their diseases.
   b) The Church promoted Galen's ideas about the human body. His work fit the Christian belief that God made human bodies and designed them to be perfect, so the Church made it central to medical teaching.
   c) The Church outlawed dissection, which meant doctors weren't allowed to investigate the human body themselves. Instead, they had to learn Galen's incorrect ideas.
2 You can choose any of the aspects, as long as you explain your answer. For example:
   The ban on dissection was most responsible for preventing medical developments during the medieval period because it prevented doctors from investigating the human body and coming up with their own medical ideas. This increased Galen's influence because it meant that doctors had little choice but to learn his ideas and were unable to identify his mistakes. The ban on dissection also made it more difficult for doctors to come up with rational explanations for disease. Rational explanations might have encouraged people to question the religious idea that disease was a punishment from God.
3 You can answer either way, as long as you explain your answer. For example:
   Astrology was significant in changing medieval attitudes to the causes of disease. Although we now know that astrology cannot be used to diagnose a patient, at the time it gave medieval people an opportunity to look beyond religious reasons for the causes of disease.

Page 9 — Natural Explanations

Knowledge and Understanding

1 a) The Four Humours Theory was created by Hippocrates in Ancient Greek times. It said that the body was made up of four humours — blood, phlegm, yellow bile and black bile. In order to maintain good health, the humours needed to be in balance.
   b) Galen thought diseases could be treated using opposites. He believed that an excessive amount of the humour that was causing a disease could be balanced out by giving the patient a food, drink, herb or spice related to the opposite humour.

2 A cold was thought to be caused by too much cold, wet phlegm, so a doctor might have told a patient with a cold to drink wine because it was considered to have hot and dry properties. Doctors thought this would balance out the humour that had caused the cold.
3 a) The miasma theory originated in Ancient Greece and Rome.
   b) The miasma theory says that bad air, which comes from anything that creates a bad smell such as human waste or dead bodies, causes disease.
   c) It was replaced by the Germ Theory in the 1860s.
4 The miasma theory encouraged people to clean the streets and do other hygienic things to prevent bad air. This sometimes helped stop the spread of disease.

Thinking Historically

1 a) Because the teachings of Galen and Hippocrates had been accepted for so long, people were unwilling to question their work. This meant that people didn't try to make their own discoveries about medicine.
   b) The Roman Catholic Church was extremely influential and powerful during the medieval period, so any medical texts approved by the Church were considered the absolute truth. This meant that it was very difficult to question any of their teachings.
   c) Medieval doctors followed Galen's ideas about anatomy because they weren't allowed to perform their own dissections. As Galen only ever dissected animals, his ideas on human anatomy were incorrect. This meant that medieval doctors had wrong ideas about the human body.
2 You can answer either way, as long as you explain your answer. For example:
   Hippocrates and Galen were the most important influences on medieval medicine in Britain. Their teachings provided two of the most popular theories about the causes of disease at the time, the Theory of the Four Humours and the miasma theory. Furthermore, their ideas were studied for centuries after their deaths, which meant their teachings were practised throughout the medieval period.

Page 11 — Islamic Medicine

Knowledge and Understanding

1 Islamic doctors kept alive a lot of medical knowledge that had been lost in the West after the fall of the Roman Empire. In the 9th century, Johannitius travelled from Baghdad to Byzantium to collect Greek medical texts and translated them into Arabic. This knowledge was then used by Avicenna to write the 'Canon of Medicine', which contained the ideas of Galen and Hippocrates, and was the most important way that classical ideas got back to Western Europe.
2 a) Albucasis wrote a book describing amputations, the removal of bladder stones and dental surgery. He also described methods for handling fractures, dislocations and the stitching of wounds.
   b) Avenzoar described the parasite that caused scabies and began to question the reliability of Galen.
   c) Ibn al-Nafis questioned Galen's ideas. He suggested that blood flows from one side of the heart to the other via the lungs and doesn't cross the septum.

Answers

3   Alchemy was important because Arabic alchemists invented useful techniques such as distillation and sublimation. They also prepared drugs such as laudanum, benzoin and camphor.

Thinking Historically

1   Similarities:
  • Both Islamic and European medical healers followed the ideas of Galen and Hippocrates in the early medieval period.
  • Religion strongly influenced both Islamic and European medicine. For example, Islam and Christianity both prohibited dissection.
  Differences:
  • Islamic doctors questioned the reliability of Galen's work in the medieval period, but European healers continued to follow Galen's teachings.
  • Islamic medicine was generally more rational and evidence-based than European medicine.

Source Analysis

1 a) This suggests that Rhazes respects Galen. Rhazes describes Galen as the 'Master' and himself as the 'disciple'. This implies that Rhazes has learnt from Galen.

  b) This suggests that Rhazes believes that some of Galen's ideas are wrong — Rhazes writes that some of Galen's 'theories' are 'erroneous'. It also suggests that even though Rhazes respects Galen, this won't prevent him from questioning Galen's teachings.

2 a) The source is useful because it was written by an Islamic scientist who appears to be familiar with the teachings of Galen. This means that it presents an informed attitude towards Galen. However, the source's usefulness is limited because it doesn't reflect attitudes towards Galen beyond the Islamic world, such as the fact that in Europe doctors continued to trust Galen's ideas until the Renaissance period.

  b) The content of the source is useful because it shows that Galen was well respected by Islamic scientists in the medieval period. The source is also useful because it shows that as early as the 9th century some Islamic scientists were beginning to question some of Galen's ideas.

Page 13 — Treating Disease

Knowledge and Understanding

1   • Pilgrimage — People believed they could be cured by travelling to holy shrines.
  • Repentance — Flagellants whipped themselves in public to show God they were sorry, as they thought disease was a punishment from God.
  • Superstitious treatments — Doctors might say certain words when providing treatment in order to make it more effective.
  • Bloodletting — If a patient was diagnosed as having 'excess blood', a small cut or leeches were used to remove blood from the body. This treatment was based on the Four Humours Theory.

  • Purging — To remove excess humours from the body, a patient was given laxatives to make them excrete fluids.
  • Purifying the air — People thought that purifying the air could prevent illness and improve health. Physicians carried posies or oranges with them when visiting patients to protect themselves from catching a disease, and during the Black Death people burned juniper, myrrh and incense to purify the air and try to prevent the disease.
  • Remedies — Early natural medicines that were made from herbs, spices, animal parts and minerals could be bought from an apothecary, a local wise woman or made at home.
  • Lucky charms — Some people used remedies based on superstitions, such as carrying lucky charms containing ingredients like 'powdered unicorn horn'.

2   Medieval doctors continued to use bloodletting because they believed strongly in the Four Humours Theory, so they were convinced that removing blood from the body would help balance the patient's humours. Their belief in the work of Galen and Hippocrates meant they overlooked the evidence that bloodletting was at best ineffective and at worst, fatal.

Thinking Historically

1   Belief in the Four Humours Theory led to treatments that removed fluids from the body, such as bloodletting and purging. These techniques were ineffective and often harmed the patient. Belief in the miasma theory meant people 'purified' the air. Physicians did this by carrying posies or oranges, and some people burnt juniper, myrrh and incense so the smoke or scent would prevent disease from spreading. These techniques were ineffective because they did nothing to address the patient's symptoms.

2 a) Evidence for — The belief that disease was a punishment from God meant prayer and repentance were common treatments.
  Evidence against — Some treatments were based on non-religious theories, such as bloodletting, which was based on the natural Four Humours Theory.

  b) Evidence for — Remedies were made from herbs, spices, animal parts and minerals.
  Evidence against — Medical treatments based on religion, such as prayer, came from spiritual beliefs rather than things found in the natural world.

  c) Evidence for — Some treatments were dangerous. For example, bloodletting caused more deaths than it prevented.
  Evidence against — Some treatments caused no harm to the patient, for example carrying a lucky charm.

3   You can answer either way for each statement, as long as you explain your answer. For example:

  a) Religion was very influential in the medieval period — prayer and repentance were two major treatments. Medieval people also sometimes went on pilgrimages or whipped themselves. They used these treatments in order to please God in the hope that he would cure them. Religious treatments dominated medicine in the medieval period.

Answers

b) Medieval people frequently used things they found around them to make medical treatments. Remedies were made from herbs, spices, animal parts and minerals. Other important treatments of the time also used things found in nature — for example, posies and oranges were used to stop 'bad air', and leeches were used for bloodletting.

c) Most medieval medical treatments tended to cause more harm than good. For example, flagellants caused harm by whipping themselves and people were more likely to die from bloodletting than to be cured by it.

Page 15 — Treating Disease

Knowledge and Understanding

1 Physician:
- Physicians were male doctors who trained at university for at least seven years, but had little practical experience.
- They read ancient texts and writings from the Islamic world.
- They used handbooks, called vademecums, and clinical observation to check their patients' conditions.
- There were fewer than 100 physicians in England in the 1300s and they were very expensive.

Apothecary:
- Apothecaries treated their patients with remedies and gave advice on how to use them.
- They were trained through apprenticeships.
- Most apothecaries were men, but there were also 'wise women' who sold herbal remedies.
- They were the most accessible and common form of treatment in medieval England.

Barber-Surgeon:
- Barber-surgeons performed minor surgical procedures.
- They also cut people's hair.

2 a) Barber-surgeon — A hernia operation was a minor procedure often performed by barber-surgeons. A poor person wouldn't be able to afford to see a university-trained surgeon.

b) Physician — They were very expensive, so only the rich could afford to see them. Rich people would choose to see a physician because they had trained for several years.

c) Hospital — The main purpose of hospitals was to care for the sick and elderly. A monastic hospital would be able to provide food, water and a warm place to stay for a sick, elderly person with no family to help them.

d) Apothecary — Apothecaries sold remedies, which would be suitable for someone with just a cough. A poor person wouldn't be able to afford a physician.

3
- Hugh and Theodoric of Lucca noticed that dressing wounds with bandages soaked in wine helped to keep wounds clean and prevent infection.
- Hugh and Theodoric of Lucca realised that pus was not a healthy sign. This was a development because most doctors at the time believed that causing wounds to pus would release toxins from the body.

- John of Arderne created a recipe for an anaesthetic in 1376 using hemlock, opium and henbane.

4 Hugh and Theodoric's work was ahead of its time because their use of practical experience and observation to make discoveries was unusual for the Middle Ages. It was something that only became more common in the Renaissance period. They also questioned Galen's teachings, which was something scientists didn't really do until after the Middle Ages.

Thinking Historically

1 a) Evidence for — Both rich and poor people could access apothecaries, hospitals and barber-surgeons.
Evidence against — Not all healthcare options were available to everyone, for example, trained physicians and surgeons were only an option for the rich.

b) Evidence for — Hospitals provided food, water and a warm place to stay. They were also more hygienic than other places. This would have helped some sick people to get better.
Evidence against — Medieval hospitals provided food, water and warmth, but they didn't treat disease. There also weren't many hospitals in medieval England, so this limited their impact.

c) Evidence for — There were only a few university-trained surgeons in the Middle Ages. The majority of operations were carried out by barber-surgeons who didn't have the same level of training. This meant that surgery could be very dangerous.
Evidence against — Surgery was generally dangerous in the medieval period because there was no way to prevent blood loss, infection or pain.

2 a) Physicians lacked practical training and experience. Because they focused on reading ancient texts rather than working with patients, they were less able to discover new treatments or make progress in medicine.

b) Apothecaries made and sold herbal remedies. Some of these remedies were written down in books called 'Herbals'. The fact that apothecaries generally just did what other apothecaries had done before them suggests that they were unlikely to make progress in treating diseases by attempting new remedies.

Page 17 — Health in Towns and Monasteries

Knowledge and Understanding

1 a) Towns didn't keep their clean water separate from waste, whereas monasteries did. In towns, water would become contaminated with waste that was thrown into rivers and by businesses like butchers, tanners and dyers throwing toxic waste into rivers and residential streets. In contrast, monasteries separated clean and dirty water by having one water supply for cooking and drinking, and another for drainage and washing. Monasteries were also built near rivers or had man-made waterways nearby so they had a source of clean water.

b) Many towns didn't have an effective method of disposing of sewage, whereas monasteries did. In towns, sewage from latrines leaked into the ground and got into wells, contaminating water. On the other hand, monasteries had latrines which were built over streams of running water which would carry sewage away without infecting their drinking water.

2 a) • Towns relied on wealthy individuals for funding, so they didn't always have the money to improve local infrastructure.
   • Monasteries were wealthy, so they could afford to build infrastructure like latrines and waterways to keep their water clean.

b) • Hundreds of people lived in towns, which made it hard to get everyone to adopt cleaner habits.
   • Monasteries had smaller populations, so it was easier to enforce rules about cleanliness and waste disposal than in towns.

c) • Towns didn't have one person in charge. This made it difficult to enforce public health measures.
   • Monasteries were led by a single, powerful leader, the abbot. He could enforce rules about cleanliness as monks were expected to obey him.

3 In the 13th century, the Great Conduit was built to bring clean water into London because the Thames was getting too toxic. In 1388, the government ordered town authorities to keep streets free of waste. As a result, towns introduced public health measures that aimed to tackle waste, sewage and pollution. For example, London and York banned dumping waste in the street and built latrines over rivers to carry sewage away. London also banned waste from being dumped in the Thames and hired carters to collect waste and take it out of the city. Many towns also ordered toxic businesses like butchers, tanners, fishmongers and dyers to move outside the city walls.

Source Analysis

1 a) The content of the source is useful for studying public health in the Middle Ages because it shows that people in cities and towns lived in unhygienic conditions as a result of waste being dumped in 'ditches, rivers, and other waters'. The source is also useful because it shows that medieval people recognised that these unhygienic conditions led to public health problems by encouraging the spread of 'intolerable diseases'. The source claims that these diseases were caused by 'corrupt and infected' air, which suggests people didn't really understand why poor hygiene led to disease and still believed in the miasma theory. The usefulness of the source's content is limited because it focuses on a public health problem that affected towns and cities. Therefore, the source cannot be used to study public health in other locations, such as monasteries or rural villages.

b) The source was written in 1388. This makes the source useful, because by this time some measures had already been taken to improve public health, such as the construction of the Great Conduit in London in the 1200s. Therefore the source suggests that earlier efforts

to improve public health had not been very successful, because towns and cities were still facing problems like 'dung and filth' in waterways in the late 1300s.

c) The purpose of the source was to prevent the spread of 'intolerable diseases' by fining people who threw waste into ditches and waterways. This is useful because it shows that people sometimes tried to do hygienic things to prevent disease and improve public health despite having mistaken beliefs about the causes of disease, such as the miasma theory. However, the usefulness of the source is limited because it doesn't provide any information about how effective this law was. In the Middle Ages, town authorities often struggled to enforce rules about public hygiene, so this law may not actually have led to significant improvements in public health.

Page 19 — The Black Death in Britain

Knowledge and Understanding

1 a) • Bubonic plague was spread by the bites of fleas from rats carried on ships.
   • Symptoms included headaches, high temperatures and pus-filled swellings on the skin.

b) • Pneumonic plague was spread by coughs and sneezes.
   • Infected people would find it painful to breathe and would cough up blood.

2 The Black Death arrived in Britain in 1348. It resulted in a huge decrease in population — it killed at least a third of British people between 1348 and 1350.

Thinking Historically

1 a) • Edward III closed Parliament in January 1349.

b) • People fasted and prayed because they thought the Black Death was a punishment from God for sinful behaviour.
   • Some people carried charms or used 'magic' potions containing arsenic to protect themselves.
   • People who believed that the plague was caused by an imbalance of the humours used purging and bloodletting.
   • Those who believed in the miasma theory carried strong smelling herbs and lit fires to 'purify' the air.

c) • People in Winchester forced the bishop to build new cemeteries outside the town because they believed that being close to the bodies of dead victims could spread the plague.
   • The people of Gloucester stopped people from entering or leaving the town. This suggests that they believed the plague was spread by human contact.

2 a) The Church encouraged people to believe that the Black Death was a punishment from God. This contributed to people using ineffective treatments, such as prayer and fasting. This belief also discouraged people from looking for practical solutions for treating the plague because they thought it was God's will.

b) People didn't have the scientific knowledge to find out what was causing the Black Death, so they were only able to base treatments on existing theories, like the Four Humours Theory and the miasma theory. These treatments were ineffective because the theories were incorrect.

Answers

c) Superstitious beliefs encouraged ineffective practices to prevent the Black Death, such as carrying charms. This did nothing to stop the disease from spreading.

3 Medieval people were powerless to stop the Black Death because they didn't have the medical knowledge to understand its causes. Many of the methods of prevention used at the time suggest they didn't realise the disease was spread by flea bites, coughs and sneezes. Instead, the methods of prevention they used show they believed in other causes, such as punishment from God or an imbalance of humours. Without the knowledge or tools to discover the real cause of the disease, medieval people had no way of being able to stop the Black Death.

4 a) The Black Death killed many people, leading to a shortage of workers. This meant workers could demand higher wages from their employers and move around to find better work. However, the 1349 Ordinance of Labourers tried to stop people moving around the country.

   b) The cost of land decreased because the Black Death meant there were fewer people. This meant some peasants were able to buy land for the first time. Some people also believe that the Black Death helped cause the Peasants' Revolt in 1381.

   c) The shortage of workers and the peasants' ability to buy land threatened the power of the elites. As a result, the government created laws, such as the 1349 Ordinance of Labourers, which tried to stop people moving around the country.

Page 21 — Exam-Style Questions

1 This question is level marked. You should look at the level descriptions on page 67 to help you mark your answer. Here are some points your answer may include:
   - Source A is useful for studying responses to the Black Death because it shows that repentance was a way that people tried to prevent the spread of the disease. Flagellants whipped themselves in order to show repentance for their sins. The account gives a lot of detail about the ritual carried out by flagellants, such as how they 'marched naked' while whipping themselves, making it very useful for studying flagellants' responses to the Black Death. However, the usefulness of the source is limited for studying responses in general because it only presents one response to the Black Death.
   - Source A is useful for studying responses to the Black Death because it shows that ineffective methods were used repeatedly. The account says that the flagellants performed the same ritual 'every night'. This reflects the fact that people in the Middle Ages rarely attempted to develop evidence-based methods of prevention and treatment, and instead continued to use methods that weren't effective in order to try to prevent and treat disease.
   - Source A is useful for this investigation because the account is from 1349, which means that it was produced during the first outbreak of the Black Death in Britain, which occurred between 1348 and 1350. Therefore, it is likely to give an accurate and reliable account of responses at this time.

   - The source is useful for studying responses to the Black Death because it was written by an English historian. This suggests that the author had good historical knowledge and so would be likely to produce a reliable account.

2 This question is level marked. You should look at the level descriptions on page 67 to help you mark your answer. Here are some points your answer may include:
   - Natural explanations of disease were important in the Middle Ages because they were very widely believed. Ideas from Galen's writings, such as the Theory of the Four Humours and the miasma theory, fit with the Christian belief that God created human bodies and made them to be perfect. Because of this, these theories were strongly supported by the Roman Catholic Church, which ensured that scholars of medicine learned them. As the Church was an extremely powerful organisation in this period, its support for natural explanations of disease meant that they were seen as the absolute truth and so were widely believed. The Church's decision to outlaw dissection also contributed to these natural explanations of disease being widely believed because it stopped doctors developing new ideas about human anatomy and meant they had to learn Galen's incorrect ideas.
   - Natural explanations of disease were important in the Middle Ages because they were incorrect and this often limited progress in the development of medicine. For example, the miasma theory taught people that disease was caused by bad air, which was proven to be incorrect in the 1860s when Pasteur developed the Germ Theory. However, because the Church supported this idea and other incorrect natural explanations, it was difficult for people to question them. Without accurate explanations for disease, people were mostly unable to develop effective methods of prevention and treatment. For example, responses to the Black Death based on the miasma theory, such as burning juniper, myrrh and incense to keep out bad air, weren't effective in preventing the disease.
   - Natural explanations of disease were important in the Middle Ages because they encouraged people to believe that disease had natural causes rather than supernatural ones. This suggested that people weren't powerless against disease and could try to take action to treat and prevent it. Some natural explanations encouraged people to do things that were effective at preventing disease. For example, the miasma theory prompted people to do hygienic things, such as cleaning the streets. However, because the explanations were wrong, they often encouraged ineffective or even harmful responses. For example, bloodletting, which was a treatment based on the Theory of the Four Humours, was ineffective and could even kill people if too much blood was removed. Therefore, while natural explanations were important for encouraging people to take action against disease, this didn't always lead to improvements in people's health.

3   This question is level marked. You should look at the level descriptions on page 67 to help you mark your answer. Here are some points your answer may include:
   - In the Middle Ages, lots of towns didn't have clean water supplies, but monasteries did. In towns, people had to get their drinking water from rivers and wells that were contaminated with toxic waste from businesses like butchers, tanners and dyers. In contrast, monasteries separated clean and dirty water. There was one water supply for cooking and drinking and another one for drainage and washing. This meant that people in monasteries didn't have to drink dirty water so they were often healthier.
   - Monasteries usually had more effective sewerage systems than towns. In monasteries, latrines were put in separate buildings, which were often built over streams of running water that carried sewage away. In towns, however, waste was often thrown into the street or into rivers, and latrines often leaked into the ground and contaminated wells. As a result, public health was worse in towns because disease could spread more easily.
   - Public health in towns was worse than in monasteries because towns had bigger populations and everybody lived more closely together. In towns, houses were usually crammed together, meaning that overcrowding and fires were common problems affecting public health. On the other hand, monasteries had small populations, so they didn't suffer from overcrowding and the problems associated with it.
   - Public health in monasteries was often better than in towns because more money was spent on infrastructure like latrine buildings and waterways. This is because monasteries were generally wealthy, whereas towns had to rely on wealthy individuals to fund these kinds of projects, so there was no guarantee that money would be spent.
   - Public health was worse in towns because it was harder to make sure people lived hygienically in towns than in monasteries. Towns didn't have one person in charge who could easily enforce public health measures. In contrast, monasteries were run by an abbot who had the power to enforce rules about cleanliness and waste disposal.

4   This question is level marked. You should look at the level descriptions on page 67 to help you mark your answer. Here are some points your answer may include:
   - The Church was very influential in the Middle Ages, so it had a significant effect on how disease was treated in this period. The Church supported the idea that disease was a punishment from God, and this encouraged people to turn to prayer and repentance in the hope that it would cure them. For example, people believed that pilgrimages to holy shrines could cure illnesses and that if a person prayed to a saint, they might intervene and stop an illness. As well as promoting supernatural ideas about the causes of disease, the Church also promoted the rational ideas of Galen by making sure that scholars of medicine learned his works. This meant that the Church played an important role in encouraging people to use treatments such as bloodletting and purging that were based on ideas like the Theory of the Four Humours. However, the Church's influence often limited the development of treatments in the Middle Ages, as it prevented people from questioning existing ideas and developing ones that might have led to more effective treatments.
   - In the Renaissance period, the Church continued to have an important influence on how disease was treated. For example, treatments such as praying and fasting, which were based on religious ideas about the causes of disease, were still used when the Great Plague struck London in 1665.
   - From the Renaissance period onwards, other institutions had a greater influence than the Church on developments in the treatment of disease. In the 16th century, the Church's influence on medicine decreased as Protestant Christianity spread to Britain. As a result, the Church no longer had so much control over medical teaching, and new medical institutions such as the College of Physicians were set up. The College of Physicians, which was founded in 1518, influenced the treatment of disease by encouraging doctors to train and to study more recent medical developments. In the modern period, other new institutions have also played an increasingly important role in developments in the treatment of disease. For example, since the late 19th century, pharmaceutical companies have been responsible for developing new drugs, such as aspirin and insulin, as well as treatments for diseases such as cancer.
   - Technological advances have been an increasingly important factor in developments in the treatment of disease from the Renaissance period onwards. For example, the invention of the printing press in the 1440s had an important influence on the treatment of disease because it meant doctors like Vesalius could print and distribute works that showed some of Galen's mistakes. This encouraged doctors to question Galen's theories and develop their own ideas, which eventually led to the development of new treatments for disease. Technology has also played a key role in enabling individuals and institutions to discover and develop new treatments. For example, the development of more advanced microscopes in the 1800s was important for Pasteur's work on the Germ Theory (published in 1861), which led to the development of new treatments, such as magic bullets, while the discovery of radiation in 1896-1898 led to the creation of radiation therapy to kill cancer cells.
   - In the 20th century, individuals played a far more important role than the Church in developments in the treatment of disease. For example, Paul Ehrlich was responsible for developing the first magic bullet, Salvarsan 606, which was used from 1911 as a treatment for syphilis. Between the 1920s and 1940s, Alexander Fleming, Howard Florey and Ernst Chain helped to develop penicillin, which is used to treat bacterial infections. These examples show that by the 20th century, the Church had very little influence on the treatment of disease and instead individual scientists played a leading role in developing new treatments.

Answers

The Beginnings of Change

Page 23 — The Renaissance
Knowledge and Understanding

1 During the medieval period, people thought that disease was caused by an imbalance in the humours. The Four Humours Theory was also popular during the Renaissance period, thanks to the rediscovery of the original writings of classical physicians like Hippocrates and Galen.

2 Protestant Christianity spread to Britain in the 16th century during the Reformation. This reduced the influence of the Catholic Church, which meant it had less control over medical teaching in the Renaissance period.

3 a) Vesalius performed dissections on criminals who had been executed.

b) Vesalius believed that successful surgery was only possible if doctors had a proper understanding of the human body. He pointed out some of Galen's mistakes and made discoveries about anatomy. For example, he showed that there were no holes in the septum of the heart.

c) 'Six Anatomical Pictures' (1538) and 'The Fabric of the Human Body' (1543).

d) He showed how important it was to dissect bodies to find out how the human body was structured. This led to dissection being used more and more in medical training. Vesalius also encouraged other doctors to question Galen.

Thinking Historically

1 a) Dissection of human bodies became an important part of medical training and research.

b) The change was due to shifting attitudes in society. In the medieval period, the Church had outlawed dissection. However, as a result of the Reformation in the 16th century, the Church's influence over medicine declined making it possible for dissection to be practised more widely. It was also due to the influence of Vesalius, who showed that dissection was important to understand the human body.

c) The printing press meant that new ideas, such as Vesalius' theories, could be spread more quickly.

d) The invention of the printing press was a technological development. It meant that books could be copied more easily, so more people had access to them.

e) Galen's teachings began to be questioned more frequently by doctors who carried out their own experiments.

f) This change was due to shifting attitudes in society as a result of the discovery of ancient books which said that anatomy and dissection were very important. Vesalius also had an influence on this change, because he showed that some of Galen's ideas were wrong and encouraged other doctors to make their own discoveries.

Page 25 — The Renaissance
Knowledge and Understanding

1 Before William Harvey, people believed that there were two kinds of blood that flowed through separate systems of blood vessels. They also thought that blood was continually formed and consumed.

2 Harvey showed that there was only one system of blood vessels and one kind of blood. He also showed that blood circulated around the body instead of being constantly formed and used up.

3 a) Paré began to use a cool salve to treat gunshot wounds instead of burning them with a red hot iron or pouring boiling oil onto them. Patients treated with a cool salve did better than those scalded with oil.

b) Before Paré, the severed blood vessels left by amputation were sealed by burning their ends with a red hot iron (cauterisation). However, Paré invented a method of tying off the vessels with threads (ligatures). This method was less painful than cauterisation, so it reduced the risk of the patient dying of shock.

Thinking Historically

1 • Vesalius used dissection to study the human anatomy more closely. Harvey developed this work by using the dissection of both humans and animals, including studying live animal hearts in action.

• Vesalius started to develop an understanding of how the human body works and produced accurate diagrams of it. Harvey built on this by adding new information about how blood circulates around the body.

2 Harvey used dissections and direct observation of living animal hearts to carry out his research. This encouraged other doctors to use similar methods. His research also helped doctors to understand anatomy better than they had before. He showed that blood wasn't continually formed and consumed, but circulated around the body. Harvey's work also proved that Vesalius had been right about the importance of dissection. His discoveries proved to other doctors that the best way to find out about the human body was to study it directly.

3 Similarities:

• All three surgeons recognised the importance of practical experience and observation. Hugh and Theodoric started using wine-soaked bandages after they observed that wine helped to prevent infection. Similarly, Paré observed that a cool salve worked better on gunshot wounds than boiling oil.

• All three surgeons made a discovery through chance. It was by chance that Hugh and Theodoric learned that bandages soaked in wine helped to keep wounds clean and prevent infection. Similarly, Paré only discovered that a cool salve helped patients with gunshot wounds because he ran out of oil during a battle.

Answers

Differences:

- Paré was an army surgeon, so his work was influenced by warfare. For example, he had to develop treatments for gunshot wounds and amputations. Hugh and Theodoric's work was not influenced by warfare.
- Although Theodoric produced textbooks recording his and Hugh's thoughts, it was difficult for them to spread their ideas because the printing press had not been invented in the 13th century. In contrast, Paré was working after the invention of the printing press so he was able to publish his ideas for other doctors to read.
- Hugh and Theodoric's experimentation was unusual for their time, the Middle Ages. However, Paré's methods of making discoveries through experimentation was more common during the Renaissance period.

4   Changes in medicine happened slowly because social attitudes were slow to change. People were reluctant to accept new ideas if they went against theories that had been taught for centuries. For example, treatments based on the Four Humours Theory, such as bloodletting, continued to be used in the period c.1500-c.1700 even though Harvey showed in the early 1600s that the reasoning behind them was incorrect. Similarly, people continued to see surgery as a low-status profession. As a result, the discoveries of surgeons like Paré weren't valued right away and so took time to bring about changes in medicine.

5   You can choose any of the individuals, as long as you explain your answer. For example:
The work of Vesalius was the most important for the development of medicine in the Renaissance period because his work encouraged other doctors to make discoveries. Vesalius was one of the first doctors to use dissection to find out more about how the human body works and his findings helped to point out some of Galen's mistakes. This influenced other doctors, such as Harvey, to use dissection to develop their own ideas, rather than just relying on Galen's writings.

Page 27 — Treatments: Continuity and Change

Knowledge and Understanding

1
- Doctors still believed in Galen's ideas. This meant they continued to use similar treatments to those used in the Middle Ages, such as bloodletting and purging.
- Seeing a doctor was still very expensive, so most people used other healers.

2   People thought that the King's touch could cure scrofula. Thousands of people with scrofula visited Charles I between 1600-1649 so he could cure them.

3   A quack was a person who had no medical knowledge, but sold medicines that didn't work and often did more harm than good. They sold their wares at fairs and markets.

4
- Councils quarantined plague victims by locking them in their houses and painting a red cross on their doors.

- Places where lots of people gathered together, such as theatres, were closed.
- The corpses of plague victims were buried in mass graves away from houses.

5   a) Carrying herbs and flowers to try to get rid of 'bad air'.
    b) Bloodletting

Thinking Historically

1   a) Both — The invention of the printing press allowed old ideas to be spread more easily. As a result, people took a greater interest in the methods used by Galen, and this meant that his treatments continued to be used in the Renaissance period. However, the printing press also meant that new ideas could be spread more easily. For example, Vesalius' discoveries about anatomy were printed and widely distributed, allowing doctors around Europe to read about his findings and learn from his discoveries. This had a limited impact though, as most people couldn't read, so new ideas only reached a small part of society.

    b) Continuity — Even though the Church had less influence in the Renaissance period, some people continued to use treatments based on religion. This is shown in people's responses to the Great Plague and the Black Death — during both outbreaks, people used prayer and fasting to try to prevent or treat the disease.

    c) Change — There were more efforts by local governments to combat the Great Plague than there had been to tackle the Black Death. New methods of prevention used by local governments during the Great Plague included quarantining plague victims.

2   Even though there had been some progress in medicine between the two plague outbreaks, the causes of the plague and how it spread were no better understood in 1665 than they had been in the 14th century. As a result, similar ineffective methods of prevention and treatment were used during the Great Plague and during the Black Death, such as wearing lucky charms and bloodletting.

Page 29 — Doctors and Surgery

Knowledge and Understanding

1   Overseas exploration brought new ingredients to Britain that could be used to treat diseases. These included guaiacum, which was believed to cure syphilis, and quinine, which was used to treat malaria. However, some of the drugs that were produced with materials from overseas may have just been advertising gimmicks.

2
- The College of Physicians was established in 1518. This improved doctors' knowledge and training by encouraging them to study recent developments in medicine.
- Doctors who trained at the College of Physicians were given a licence. This separated them from quack doctors and helped to improve standards.
- New weapons like cannons and guns were used in warfare. This meant surgeons learnt how to treat new types of injuries.
- Dissections became a key part of medical training in the 1700s. This enabled doctors to see how the body actually worked and gave them a greater understanding of human anatomy.

Answers

Thinking Historically

1 a) War led to the development of new surgical treatments. New weapons like cannons and guns were developed, which led to new types of injuries. This meant surgeons had to come up with new treatments for injuries they hadn't seen before.

b) Individuals developed new surgical techniques during this period. For example, Paré improved the treatment of amputations. His method of tying off blood vessels with ligatures reduced the risk of the patient dying of shock. John Hunter introduced a new way to treat an aneurysm in the leg. He tied off the blood vessel to encourage blood to flow through the other vessels. This prevented the patient having to have their leg amputated.

c) The invention of the printing press in the 1440s meant surgeons were better able to communicate their findings. For example, Paré published his ideas and this enabled British surgeons to use his methods. Over time this helped to improve surgical techniques.

d) The creation of the London College of Surgeons in 1800 helped to improve standards in surgery. The College set training standards for surgeons which improved their surgical knowledge and techniques. This helped surgeons gain the same high status as doctors.

2 You can choose any of the factors, as long as you explain your answer. For example:
Communication was the most important factor in the development of surgery in the period c.1500-c.1800. This is because the invention of printing meant that it was possible for surgeons to share their work widely and learn from one another's discoveries. Without the improvement in communication brought about by the invention of printing, the discoveries made by individuals and as a result of war might not have become so widely known. This would have slowed down the development of surgery or might even have prevented some developments from happening at all.

Source Analysis

1 a) The source was written by John Hunter, one of the most influential figures in surgery during the 1700s. This makes the source useful for studying surgery in the 1700s because it is likely to provide a reliable and well-informed insight into what surgery was like during this period.

b) The content of the source is useful for studying surgery in the 1700s because it reflects the influence of warfare on surgery in this period. Hunter says that his time as an army surgeon gave him 'extensive opportunities of attending to gunshot wounds', and that he used these opportunities to come up with improvements to existing surgical methods. The content of the source is also useful because it demonstrates that in the 18th century some surgeons were using scientific methods in order to come up with more effective techniques. For example, Hunter says that his work is based on 'observations'. This reflects Hunter's emphasis on the importance of good scientific habits, such as learning as much about the body as possible to understand illness, experimenting to find better ways to treat disease, and testing treatments before using them.

c) Hunter says that the purpose of the source is 'the improvement of surgery'. This makes the source useful because it shows that by the 18th century some surgeons were deliberately trying to identify 'errors and defects' in surgery and trying to fix them. This represents a big shift from the Middle Ages, when most doctors tended to rely on the ideas of classical writers like Galen without questioning them. The purpose of the source also makes it useful because it demonstrates that in the 18th century surgeons used books in order to try and spread new ideas. However, the usefulness of the source is limited because it doesn't provide any information about how much Hunter's ideas actually influenced other surgeons in the 1700s.

Page 31 — Hospitals
Knowledge and Understanding

1 a) Several charity hospitals opened from the early 18th century, including the Middlesex Infirmary, The London Hospital and Guy's Hospital. They were funded by the rich and offered largely free treatment to the poor. Some charity hospitals specialised in treating certain illnesses, or providing somewhere for mothers to give birth. However, only those who were likely to recover were admitted, due to the lack of space and the risk of contagious illnesses spreading. The 'deserving' poor had a greater chance of being admitted to charity hospitals.

b) Dispensaries offered non-residential medical care to poor people. Medicines and non-surgical services from people like dentists and midwives were provided for free.

c) Most poor people were treated in workhouses. These were large buildings that people went to if they could no longer look after themselves. Conditions in workhouses were often poor, but from the 1850s there was a partially successful movement to improve conditions in workhouse infirmaries.

d) Medical school hospitals were founded in the 19th century. These included Charing Cross Hospital, University College Hospital and King's College Hospital. These hospitals were used to train doctors and conduct scientific research.

e) Cottage hospitals opened from the 1860s. They were run by GPs and provided care to people in rural areas.

Thinking Historically

1 a) • Medieval hospitals — There were relatively few hospitals.
• Hospitals in c.1700-c.1900 — Many more hospitals were built in this period.

b) • Medieval hospitals — Hospitals were run by the Church.
• Hospitals in c.1700-c.1900 — Hospitals were run by local authorities, universities and GPs.

c) • Medieval hospitals — Hospitals provided sick and elderly people with a warm place to stay as well as food and clean water.
• Hospitals in c.1700-c.1900 — Most hospitals focused on treating disease.

d) • Medieval hospitals — Hospitals were hygienic. Waste was kept separate from clean water and they had good sewerage systems.
• Hospitals in c.1700-c.1900 — Hospitals became cleaner and more hygienic during this period.

Source Analysis

1 Here are some points your answer may include:
• The source suggests that Florence Nightingale improved the relationship between female nurses and the army. In the image, Nightingale can be seen working alongside a male army officer. This suggests that female nurses were able to work with soldiers, despite the army's opposition to female nurses before Nightingale went to Scutari.
• The source suggests that Nightingale wanted her patients to be well fed. It shows a nurse holding a bowl out to a patient, which suggests that the nurse is feeding the patient.
• The source suggests that Nightingale made sure that wards were clean and hygienic. In the image, the ward is very tidy and the floor is clean.

2 This makes the source useful for an investigation into the development of hospitals in the 19th century because the author is likely to have visited Scutari Hospital himself or based his drawing on first-hand accounts from people in Crimea who had visited the hospital. Therefore the source probably gives quite an accurate representation of what the hospital was like after Florence Nightingale took over there.

Page 33 — Jenner and Vaccination

Knowledge and Understanding

1 Smallpox was originally prevented through a process called inoculation. A cut was made in a patient's arm and this was soaked in pus from the swelling of somebody who already had a mild form of smallpox.

2 It didn't involve infecting the patient with smallpox, which could sometimes be deadly.

3 • 1796 — Jenner infected James Phipps with cowpox pus from the sores of Sarah Nelmes. He then infected Phipps with smallpox and Phipps didn't catch the disease.
• 1798 — Jenner published his findings about the smallpox vaccination.
• 1802 — Parliament approved of Jenner's vaccination and gave him £10,000 to open a clinic.
• 1840 — The smallpox vaccination was made free for infants.
• 1853 — The vaccination was made compulsory.

Thinking Historically

1 • Some doctors who gave the old smallpox inoculation had a negative attitude towards Jenner's vaccination because they saw it as a threat to their livelihood.
• Many people were concerned about the safety of the vaccination — they worried about giving themselves a disease from cows.

• Some people opposed the vaccination because they didn't believe it worked well. For example, a doctor called William Woodville claimed the vaccination was little better than inoculation after several smallpox deaths occurred at his hospital.
• Some opposition to the vaccination was a result of attitudes towards the role that the government should play in people's lives. For example, several groups opposed the decision to make the vaccination compulsory in 1853 because they didn't like the idea of the government telling them what to do.

2 a) • They approved of Jenner's discovery and gave him £10,000 to open a vaccination clinic in 1802.
• They gave Jenner a further £20,000 a few years later.
• They made the vaccination free for infants in 1840 and then made it compulsory in 1853.

b) • Lady Mary Wortley Montagu learned about the method of inoculation in Turkey and promoted it in Britain. Her work showed that smallpox could be prevented.
• Edward Jenner used careful scientific methods to demonstrate that people who had had cowpox didn't get smallpox. He used an experiment to show that he could prevent people from catching smallpox by injecting them with pus from the sores of people suffering from cowpox.

3 You can answer either way, as long as you explain your answer. For example:
Parliament was more important to the success of the smallpox vaccination. Although Jenner came up with the idea, it was Parliament that ensured the vaccination became widely used. Parliament funded a vaccination clinic, gave Jenner a further £20,000 a few years later and eventually made the smallpox vaccination compulsory in 1853. Without this support from Parliament, it is unlikely that Jenner's vaccination would have reached so many people and succeeded in bringing about a big fall in the number of smallpox cases in Britain.

4 • Jenner and Harvey both carried out experiments while developing their ideas. Jenner tested his smallpox vaccination on James Phipps, while Harvey studied living animal hearts and applied his findings to humans.
• Both men's work developed ideas that already existed. Jenner's vaccination improved Montagu's method of inoculation, while Harvey built on the work of Vesalius, who had demonstrated the importance of dissection and begun to improve people's understanding of anatomy.
• Both men struggled to get their work accepted. Jenner faced resistance from the public and doctors when he introduced his vaccination. Harvey's idea that blood circulates around the body instead of being continually formed and consumed wasn't believed by many doctors at first. As a result, they continued to use bloodletting even though Harvey had shown the reasoning behind it to be wrong.

Answers

Page 35 — Exam-Style Questions

1 This question is level marked. You should look at the level descriptions on page 67 to help you mark your answer. Here are some points your answer may include:

- Source A is useful for studying Jenner's work on vaccination because it gives an insight into people's fears about the smallpox vaccination. In the cartoon, a grotesque cow-like creature with big jaws and jagged teeth represents vaccination. The animal's threatening appearance reflects the fact that many people in the early 19th century saw vaccination as something frightening and dangerous. The animal is covered in sores and the names of diseases, and the infants that it excretes have horns and tails. This suggests that people's fear of vaccination was based on concerns that it could cause health problems rather than preventing them. This fear may have come about because the careful scientific methods Jenner used to develop vaccination were unusual at the time, so most people probably didn't understand that they meant his vaccination could be trusted. This is suggested in the image by the portrayal of Jenner feeding children to the threatening cow-like creature. This creates the impression that, far from trying to protect the public, Jenner doesn't care about people's safety at all.

- Source A is useful because it reflects the public's attitude towards the government's support for Jenner's work. The source was produced in 1802 when Parliament gave Jenner £10,000 to open a vaccination clinic, an event that is represented in the image by the document in Jenner's back pocket with the figure of £10,000 on it. The negative portrayal of Jenner in the image, with horns and a tail, and the image's focus on the supposed dangers of vaccination, suggest that the artist wanted to criticise Parliament's decision to fund Jenner's work. Cartoons like Source A often reflect wider public opinion, so the cartoonist may be expressing broader public opposition to Parliament's support for Jenner.

- Source A is useful for an investigation into Jenner's work on vaccination because it was produced in 1802. This was just four years after Jenner published his findings about the smallpox vaccination in 1798 and is the same year that Jenner received backing from the government. This means the source reflects the immediate response to Jenner's work on vaccination. However, the date of the source means that it is not useful for studying the longer-term significance of Jenner's work. For example, it does not reflect the fact that the smallpox vaccination became free for infants in 1840 and compulsory in 1853, nor does it reflect the long-term success of the vaccination in reducing the number of smallpox cases in Britain.

2 This question is level marked. You should look at the level descriptions on page 67 to help you mark your answer. Here are some points your answer may include:

- Harvey's work was important for the development of medicine because it improved doctors' understanding of the human body. Harvey showed that blood circulates around the body, rather than being continually formed and consumed. This gave doctors a new understanding of how the body works, changing their understanding of anatomy.

- Harvey's work was important because it showed that Galen's idea that there were two different kinds of blood flowing through separate systems of blood vessels was wrong. Discoveries like this that identified Galen's mistakes encouraged doctors to base their ideas on observation and not just on the books of ancient doctors. This new approach was vital for the development of new ideas in medicine.

- Harvey's work was important because, like Vesalius, he used human dissection as well as studying animals. Using dissection to study human bodies improved doctors' understanding of the body and led to important developments in medicine.

- Harvey studied at Padua University in Italy. This was important because major new discoveries were being made at universities in France and Italy during the Renaissance, such as Vesalius' discovery that there were no holes in the septum of the heart. Harvey was able to bring some of these ideas back to Britain.

- Harvey's work was more important in the long term than the short term because it took a long time to make an impact. For example, bloodletting continued as a treatment in the Renaissance period even though Harvey had shown that it was based on a mistaken belief.

3 This question is level marked. You should look at the level descriptions on page 67 to help you mark your answer. Here are some points your answer may include:

- People did not know what caused either the Black Death or the Great Plague. Both epidemics were believed by many to be caused by miasma or were seen as a punishment from God. As a result, in both periods people tried to purify the air and prayed in an attempt to prevent the disease.

- Superstition influenced attempts to prevent both the Black Death and the Great Plague. People tried to prevent the Black Death by carrying charms or using magic potions containing arsenic. Similarly, during the Great Plague people wore lucky charms and amulets to prevent the disease. In both periods, these measures based on superstition were ineffective at preventing the disease.

- During both the Black Death and the Great Plague, local government attempts at prevention were limited and ultimately ineffective. During the Black Death, Winchester built cemeteries for plague victims away from houses, while Gloucester attempted to avoid the Black Death by shutting itself off from the outside world. Similar techniques were used during the Great Plague — local councils quarantined plague victims and placed dead victims' bodies in mass graves away from houses.

- There was no national government response to either the Black Death or the Great Plague. King Edward III closed Parliament in January 1349 in response to the Black Death, but did nothing to prevent the disease elsewhere in the country. Likewise, there was no national government response to the Great Plague.

Answers

4 This question is level marked. You should look at the level descriptions on page 67 to help you mark your answer. Here are some points your answer may include:

- In the Middle Ages, the Church played a more important role than individuals in understanding the causes of disease. The Church made sure that scholars of medicine learnt the ideas of Hippocrates and Galen, many of which were incorrect. For example, miasma theory taught that disease was caused by bad air and the Four Humours Theory argued that disease was caused by an imbalance of the humours. Because the Church was so influential it was hard for people to question these ideas around the causes of disease. Also, because the Church outlawed dissection, it was very difficult for individuals to develop their own ideas about the human body and the causes of disease. Therefore, in the Middle Ages, the Church limited progress in understanding the causes of disease, because the ideas it promoted were incorrect and individuals were unable to question them.

- In the Renaissance period, the influence of the Church over medicine began to decline, and as a result the role of individuals became increasingly important in understanding the causes of disease. In the mid-16th century, Vesalius used human dissection to correct some of Galen's mistakes. For example, he showed that there were no holes in the septum of the heart. In the 17th century, the work of William Harvey showed that there was only one kind of blood which circulated around the body. This disproved Galen's belief that there were two kinds of blood flowing in separate systems. The work of individuals like Vesalius and Harvey was important because it gave people a more accurate picture of how the human body worked, which was essential for achieving a better understanding of the causes of disease. However, it took a long time for their work to have an impact because people continued to believe in older ideas about the causes of disease, such as the Four Humours Theory.

- The impact of individuals' ideas on people's understanding of the causes of disease relied on improvements in communication. Without developments like the invention of the printing press, it is unlikely that individuals like Vesalius and Harvey would have been able to spread their ideas as widely as they did.

- The work of individuals was a very important factor in the development of ideas about the causes of disease in the 19th century. For example, in 1861 Louis Pasteur published the Germ Theory, which showed that some germs cause disease. Before his discovery, people still believed in the miasma theory, which blamed disease on 'bad air'. Although people had been aware of the existence of germs since the 17th century, they thought that they were caused by disease. Another individual, Robert Koch, built on the Germ Theory by linking specific diseases, such as anthrax and tuberculosis, to the microbes that caused them. Germ Theory, combined with Koch's scientific techniques, gave other microbe hunters the knowledge to make more discoveries about the causes of disease. For example, Edwin Klebs discovered the diphtheria germ in 1883.

- Individuals also played a key role in improving people's understanding of the causes of disease in towns and cities in the 19th century. For example, in 1842 Edwin Chadwick published a report which showed that there was a link between poor living conditions in towns and health problems. In 1853-54, John Snow developed this idea further when he showed that cholera was caused by contaminated water. He noticed that cholera victims in the Broad Street area of London were using the same water pump, so he removed the handle from the pump, and this ended the cholera outbreak.

- Research organisations and institutions have played an important role in improving understanding of the causes of disease since the Renaissance period. The College of Physicians, which was set up in 1518, has helped to improve doctors' understanding of the causes of disease by ensuring that they study recent medical developments as part of their training. Since the 19th century, hospitals founded alongside universities or medical schools have also helped doctors to develop their understanding of the causes of disease by acting as training schools for doctors or by conducting scientific research.

- Technology has been an important factor in understanding the causes of disease because it has helped many individuals to make their discoveries. For example, Pasteur's work on the Germ Theory was made possible by the development of more powerful microscopes during the 1800s. These new microscopes helped Pasteur to study microbes because they enabled him see clearer images of germs with a lot less light distortion.

A Revolution in Medicine

Page 37 — The Germ Theory
Knowledge and Understanding

1 a) The belief that germs were created by decaying matter, such as human waste or rotting food. It made people think that disease caused germs.
  b) The theory that microbes in the air cause decay and that some germs cause disease.

2 Pasteur showed that sterilised water that was kept in a closed flask stayed sterile, whereas sterilised water in an open flask bred germs. This suggested that there were germs in the air which entered the open flask.

3 a) He identified the anthrax bacteria.
  b) He found the bacteria that cause septicaemia.
  c) He found the bacteria that cause tuberculosis.
  d) He found the bacteria that cause cholera.

Answers

4
- Agar jelly to create solid cultures and breed bacteria.
- Dyes to stain bacteria so they were more visible under a microscope.
- Photography to record his findings.
- Advanced microscopes that provided clearer images of small objects.

Thinking Historically

1   You can answer either way, as long as you explain your answer. For example:
The role of individuals was more important than the role of new technology in the development of the Germ Theory. Although the development of more advanced microscopes during the 1800s made it easier for Pasteur to observe germs, it was Pasteur's individual ideas and techniques that led to the breakthrough in understanding the causes of disease. For example, Pasteur came up with an experiment to prove the presence of germs in the air, and he went on to prove the link between germs and disease by demonstrating in 1867 that germs caused a disease in silkworms. The importance of Pasteur as an individual is highlighted by the fact that scientists had been aware of microbes since the 17th century, but no-one realised their significance in causing disease until Pasteur investigated the souring of sugar beet in the mid-19th century.

2 a) The Germ Theory was important because it correctly explained a major cause of disease. This helped doctors and scientists to develop effective methods of prevention and treatment for a range of diseases, and also contributed to the development of surgery by helping inspire Joseph Lister to develop antiseptics. In addition, the Germ Theory led to improvements in public health because it linked disease to poor living conditions, and this put pressure on the government to pass the 1875 Public Health Act.

   b) The smallpox vaccination was important because it was one of the first effective methods of preventing disease. The vaccination was safer than the previous method of inoculation and it contributed to a big fall in deaths from smallpox, which had been one of the most deadly diseases in the 1700s. The vaccination was also important because Jenner developed it by using an experiment. This was important because in the late 18th century it was still unusual for doctors to test their theories.

3   You can answer either way, as long as you explain your answer. For example:
The Germ Theory was more important for the development of medicine because it led to huge progress in surgery, public health and the prevention and treatment of disease. In contrast, the smallpox vaccination did not lead directly to other significant developments in medicine because Jenner didn't understand why the vaccination worked. It was only after the Germ Theory was developed that scientists were able to develop vaccinations that prevented other diseases.

Page 39 — The Fight against Germs

Knowledge and Understanding

1
- chicken cholera
- anthrax
- rabies

2 a) Edwin Klebs discovered the diphtheria germ in 1883.
   b) Friedrich Loeffler cultured the diphtheria germ and found that its effect on people was due to a toxin it produced.
   c) In 1891, Emil von Behring produced an antitoxin from the blood of animals that had just recovered from diphtheria. This could be used to reduce the effect of the disease.
   d) Ronald Ross discovered how malaria is transmitted. In 1902 he received the Nobel Prize for his work.

3   Magic bullets are synthetic antibodies. They are called 'magic bullets' because they only attack specific microbes.

4
- 1889 — Ehrlich begins to research chemicals that could act as synthetic antibodies.
- 1905 — The bacteria that causes syphilis is identified. Ehrlich and his team decide to search for an arsenic compound that is a magic bullet for syphilis.
- 1909 — Sahachiro Hata joins Ehrlich's team and rechecks the results. He notices that compound number 606 appears to work.
- 1911 — Salvarsan 606 is used on a human for the first time.

Thinking Historically

1 a) The work of Pasteur and other individuals on his team was important to the development of new vaccines because they worked out that attenuated cholera could make chickens immune to the disease and used this breakthrough to create vaccines for other diseases, such as anthrax and rabies. Pasteur's work on vaccines was inspired by his personal and political rivalry with Robert Koch.
   b) Chance led to the discovery of a vaccine for chicken cholera by Pasteur and his team. Pasteur's assistant, Charles Chamberland, injected some chickens with a cholera culture that had been weakened by being accidentally left out on a desk. This chance mistake led to the discovery that the chickens became immune to cholera after being exposed to a weakened form of the bacteria.

2   You can choose either of the factors, as long as you explain your answer. For example:
Individuals were the most important factor for the development of new vaccines. While chance gave Pasteur and his team an important starting point for the creation of the chicken cholera vaccine, it was individuals who recognised the significance of Chamberland's chance discovery and worked out how to apply it to other diseases.

Answers

3   Koch was important for the development of medicine because he identified the bacteria that cause a number of different diseases, such as anthrax, septicaemia, tuberculosis and cholera. These discoveries were important because they led to breakthroughs in the prevention of disease. For example, Pasteur and his team built on Koch's discovery of the anthrax bacteria by developing a vaccine for this disease. In addition, Koch's scientific techniques, such as using dyes to stain bacteria to make them more visible, were important for the development of medicine because they made microbe hunting easier. Koch's methods were used by other scientists to make important medical breakthroughs such as the development of a treatment for diphtheria and the discovery of how malaria is transmitted.

4   There was only slow progress in the treatment of disease between the 1860s and the 1940s because scientists still needed to work out how to use the Germ Theory to develop new treatments for diseases, and this could take a very long time. For example, the diphtheria germ was discovered in 1883, but it wasn't until eight years later in 1891 that Emil von Behring produced an antitoxin that could be used to reduce the effect of the disease. Similarly, it took Paul Ehrlich and his team four years to identify a magic bullet that could treat syphilis, and it was a further two years before they were able to use it on humans. It wasn't until the pharmaceutical industry took off in the 1940s that the Germ Theory began to lead to greater changes in the treatment of disease.

Page 41 — Anaesthetics

Knowledge and Understanding

1   They stop patients feeling pain during surgery. This is important because patients can die from the trauma of extreme pain.

2 a) A Professor of Midwifery who experimented with various chemicals in order to try and find a safe alternative to ether that women could take during childbirth. In 1847 he discovered that chloroform was an effective anaesthetic and was easier to use than ether. After Queen Victoria used chloroform during childbirth in 1853 it became widely used in operating theatres and to reduce pain in childbirth.

b) A British chemist who identified nitrous oxide (laughing gas) as a possible anaesthetic in 1799. He was ignored by surgeons at the time.

c) An American doctor who discovered that ether could be used as an anaesthetic in 1842. His work had little impact because he didn't publish his findings.

d) An American dentist who used nitrous oxide in a public demonstration in 1845. He chose a patient who was unaffected by nitrous oxide and so he was ignored.

e) In 1884, he investigated the use of cocaine as a local anaesthetic.

f) An American dental surgeon who carried out the first public demonstration of ether as an anaesthetic in 1846.

3 a) It doesn't work on everyone.

b) It's an irritant and is also fairly explosive.

c) It's addictive.

4   1846-1870 is known as the 'Black Period' of surgery because the death rate from operations increased as the development of anaesthetics enabled surgeons to attempt longer and more complicated procedures. The longer operating times meant there was a great risk of infection.

Thinking Historically

1   You can choose any of the individuals, as long as you explain your answer. For example:
James Simpson made the most important contribution to the development of anaesthetics because he discovered the effects of chloroform, which was a relatively safe anaesthetic. This was more important than the work of doctors like Crawford Long, William Morton and William Halsted on ether and cocaine because these anaesthetics had serious drawbacks — ether is fairly explosive and cocaine is highly addictive. Simpson's contribution was more important than those of Humphry Davy and Horace Wells because their work on nitrous oxide was ignored by surgeons, whereas Simpson's anaesthetic became widely used in operating theatres and during childbirth.

2   Here are some points your answer may include:
Positive effect:
- Anaesthetics made patients easier to operate on, which meant surgeons didn't have to rush their procedures.
- Developments in anaesthetics meant that more complicated surgeries could be carried out.

Negative effect:
- Anaesthetics led to more complex surgeries, which caused increased death rates because surgeons were more ambitious.
- Anaesthetics led to longer operating times, which meant that death rates from infection increased.

3 a) Continuity — Surgeons still didn't know that clean clothes could prevent infection, so they often wore the same dirty coats for years.

b) Change — Different anaesthetics were tested during this period to find a safe alternative to natural drugs like alcohol and opium. After 1853, chloroform became widely used in operating theatres.

c) Continuity — Operations continued to be carried out in unhygienic locations, such as people's homes.

d) Change — The development of effective anaesthetics meant that operations became longer. This was because it was easier for surgeons to operate on unconscious patients, so they didn't have to rush and could attempt more complex procedures.

Answers

Page 43 — Antiseptics

Knowledge and Understanding

1 Antiseptic surgical methods aim to kill germs, whereas aseptic surgical methods aim to prevent germs from getting near the wound.

2 a) Semmelweis showed doctors that they could reduce the spread of infection by washing their hands with chloride of lime.

b) Lister saw carbolic acid sprays being used in sewage works to keep down the smell. He tried this in his operating theatre in the early 1860s and infection rates fell.

c) When Lister heard about the Germ Theory, he realised that germs could be on objects in the operating theatre, so he starting using carbolic acid to kill the germs on things like surgical instruments and bandages.

3 It was unpleasant to get on your skin or breathe in, so doctors were opposed to using it.

4 • They sterilise instruments with high temperature steam.
  • They sterilise their hands before entering the operating theatre.
  • They wear sterilised gowns, masks, gloves and hats.
  • They keep operating theatres clean and fill them with sterile air.

Thinking Historically

1 • They made surgery more hygienic, which reduced death rates from around 50% in 1864-66 to 15% in 1867-70.
  • They allowed surgeons to operate with less fear of patients dying from infection.
  • They led to a tenfold increase in the number of operations between 1867 and 1912.

2 You can choose any of the factors, as long as you explain your answer. For example:
Individuals were the most important factor in the development of surgery in the period c.1800-c.1900. Chance mainly played a negative role in this period. For example, chance contributed to nitrous oxide being ignored as a possible anaesthetic because Horace Wells had the bad luck to pick a patient who was unaffected by the drug when he held a public demonstration in 1845. Communication played an important role in encouraging surgeons to adopt new techniques. For example, Lister promoted the use of carbolic spray in his well-publicised operation at King's College Hospital in 1877. However, without Lister's experimentation with carbolic acid in the 1860s, there would have been no surgical breakthrough to promote. This shows that the role of communication relied on the work done by individuals such as Lister. Therefore, individuals were more important than communication in the development of surgery during this period.

Source Analysis

1 The date of the source makes it useful for studying surgery in the 19th century because it was published after effective anaesthetics and antiseptics had been developed. For example, James Simpson discovered that chloroform was an effective anaesthetic in 1847, and Joseph Lister began using a carbolic spray in operating theatres and putting carbolic acid on instruments and bandages in the 1860s. Therefore, the source is likely to reflect the way these developments had affected surgery by the 1880s.

2 • The content of the source is useful because it reflects the development of antiseptics in the 19th century. The image shows a carbolic acid spray on the table on the left. This reflects the growing use of antiseptics in surgery from the 1860s onwards, thanks to the work of Joseph Lister.
  • The content of the source is useful because it shows the growing use of anaesthetics during this period. In the source, the patient is receiving anaesthetic through a mask. This reflects the development of increasingly safe and effective anaesthetics during the 19th century to replace natural drugs like alcohol, opium and mandrake. In particular, this is likely to reflect the use of chloroform, which became widely used in operating theatres after Queen Victoria used it during childbirth in 1853.

Page 45 — Public Health

Knowledge and Understanding

1 a) As a result of the industrial revolution, lots of people moved to towns and cities to work in factories. This affected public health because towns and cities grew so quickly that good housing couldn't be built fast enough — houses were built too close together, with little outside space and poor ventilation.

b) Living conditions were often unhygienic and overcrowding was a big problem. Families with four or more children often lived in a single room and the poorest lived in cellars. This affected public health because it was easy for diseases like cholera to spread in these conditions.

c) Most houses had no bathroom, and instead people shared an outside privy. Each privy was built above a cesspit, and waste from these cesspits was either thrown into rivers or piled up for the rain to wash away. The lack of good sewerage systems made it easier for diseases to spread.

d) Water companies set up water pumps in the streets which were shared between many houses. This led to public health problems because the water supplies for the pumps were often contaminated by waste from cesspits or from rivers.

2 Cholera is a disease that is caused by infected sewage entering drinking water. It causes extreme diarrhoea, which can lead to death. It reached Britain in 1831 and caused four epidemics between 1832 and 1866. It killed tens of thousands of people in Britain during the 19th century.

3 Chadwick found that living conditions in towns were worse for people's health than conditions in the countryside. Therefore he recommended that the government should pass laws for proper drainage and sewerage systems, funded by local taxes.

4   • The Act set up a central Board of Health, but this was dismantled in 1858.
    • The Act allowed any town to set up its own local board of health as long as the town's taxpayers agreed. However, very few towns chose to do this, and those that did often refused to spend any money to improve conditions.

5   In 1853-54 John Snow studied a cholera outbreak in the Broad Street area of London and noticed that the victims all used the same water pump. When he removed the handle from the pump, the outbreak ended. This was important for public health because it showed that there was a connection between contaminated water and cholera.

Source Analysis

1 a) This suggests that contaminated water was still killing people in 1866, and may reflect the fact that Britain suffered its fourth cholera epidemic in 1865-66. It also suggests that by 1866 people recognised the link between contaminated water and deadly diseases like cholera, which may reflect the influence of John Snow's work on the Broad Street cholera outbreak of 1853-54.

  b) The caption suggests that the artist blames the government for the deaths caused by contaminated water. This suggests that by 1866 some people thought that the government should do more to protect people from public health problems like contaminated water.

2   The source was published in 1866. This makes the source useful for an investigation into public health in the 19th century because it indicates that by the 1860s there had been little progress in solving the public health problem of contaminated water causing deadly diseases. This suggests that the work of Edwin Chadwick and John Snow, and the introduction of the 1848 Public Health Act had little immediate impact on public health.

Page 47 — Public Health

Knowledge and Understanding

1   The 'Great Stink' was a bad smell caused by pollution in the River Thames in the summer of 1858. The smell developed when hot weather caused the river's water level to drop and bacteria to grow in the waste that drained into the Thames.

2   • Evidence from Chadwick and Snow, and Pasteur's Germ Theory, suggested that cleaning towns could stop the spread of disease. This made people want the government to do more to make sure towns were clean.
    • In 1867, the Second Reform Act was passed which gave the vote to one million more men, most of whom were industrial workers. This meant that, for the first time, politicians had to pay attention to workers in order to stay in power. Therefore, workers were able to put pressure on the government to address their concerns about health.

  • Reformers pushed the government to become more involved in public health. For example, William Farr, a statistician who recorded causes of death, used his statistics to press for reforms in areas where death rates were high.

3   The 1875 Public Health Act was compulsory, whereas the one in 1848 said that towns could choose whether to set up a health board or spend money on improving conditions.

4 a) Councils appointed health and sanitary inspectors who made sure laws on water supplies and hygiene were followed. It also made councils maintain sewerage systems and keep their towns' streets clean.

  b) It allowed local councils to buy slums with poor living conditions and turn them into houses that were built to a government-approved standard.

Thinking Historically

1   The 'Great Stink' was important for the improvement of public health because it led to the government appointing Joseph Bazalgette to build a new sewer system in London. These sewers transported waste that was normally dumped in the Thames away from heavily populated areas. This meant that they improved public health by cleaning up London's drinking water and preventing the spread of waterborne diseases like cholera.

2   You can choose any of the factors, as long as you explain your answer. For example:
  Chance was the most important factor in ending cholera outbreaks in London. The government and individuals played an important role because the government took the decision that London needed new sewers, and Joseph Bazalgette designed the new sewer system. However, chance was a more important factor because when work started on the project, neither the government nor Bazalgette fully understood how cholera spread. This meant that their aim was to prevent another 'Great Stink' from the Thames, rather than to clean up London's drinking water. Therefore, it was only by chance that their solution to the problem of bad smells also happened to tackle the cause of cholera and prevent future outbreaks of the disease.

3   For:
  • Edwin Chadwick played an important role in improving public health because his 1842 report demonstrated that living conditions in towns were worse for people's health than conditions in the countryside. He made recommendations that would improve public health, such as using local taxes to fund proper drainage and sewerage systems.
  • John Snow showed that there was a connection between contaminated water and cholera. This was important for improving public health because it helped people to understand why the unhygienic conditions in towns led to public health problems.

Answers

- Joseph Bazalgette played an important role in improving public health because he built a new sewer system in London to transport waste away from heavily populated areas to the Thames Estuary. This cleaned up London's drinking water, preventing outbreaks of waterborne diseases like cholera.
- William Farr helped to improve public health by using his statistics on causes of death to push for reforms in areas where death rates were high.
- The work of Louis Pasteur was important in improving public health because his Germ Theory linked disease to poor living conditions like contaminated water. This encouraged people to take action to tackle public health problems.

Against:
- The direct impact that some individuals had on public health was limited. For example, Chadwick's 1842 report encouraged the government to pass the 1848 Public Health Act, which set up a central Board of Health and allowed towns to set up their own local boards of health. However, this didn't improve public health significantly because very few towns chose to set up health boards and the central Board of Health was dismantled in 1858.
- Changing attitudes were an important factor in improving public health. For most of the 19th century, people believed in a laissez-faire style of government, and so there was little government action to tackle public health problems. It was only when this attitude began to change that the government took action to improve public health.
- The government played a very important role in improving public health in the 19th century, because it passed the 1875 Public Health Act. This Act helped to tackle many public health problems because it forced councils to keep town streets clean, maintain sewerage systems and appoint health inspectors and sanitary inspectors to make sure that laws on things like water supplies and hygiene were followed.

Page 49 — Exam-Style Questions

1 This question is level marked. You should look at the level descriptions on page 67 to help you mark your answer. Here are some points your answer may include:
- Source A is useful for studying public health in 19th-century Britain because it was written in 1842 by Edwin Chadwick, a social reformer who led a team of commissioners that travelled the country to find out what life was like for poor people. This means Chadwick had a good understanding of what public health was like in the mid-19th century. As a result, the source is likely to provide an accurate view of what public health was like before the government moved away from its laissez-faire approach in the later 19th century.
- Source A is useful because it gives an insight into people's understanding of the causes of poor public health in the 1840s. Chadwick argues that overcrowding and dirty living conditions contribute

to the spread of disease. This shows that even before the Germ Theory was developed by Pasteur in 1861, people recognised that poor living conditions in towns were contributing to poor public health. However, Chadwick also claims that disease is caused by 'atmospheric impurities', which suggests he believed in the miasma theory. This reflects the fact that in the 1840s people still didn't understand why problems like dirty living conditions caused poor public health. It was only in the 1860s when Pasteur's Germ Theory confirmed John Snow's findings about the link between cholera and contaminated water that people began to gain a more accurate understanding of the causes of poor public health.
- The usefulness of Source A is limited for studying how public health problems were eventually tackled in the 19th century. In the report, Chadwick recommends removing waste from living areas and improving water and drainage systems in order to improve public health. However, it took a very long time for the government to enforce measures like the ones Chadwick suggests. Six years after Chadwick published his report, the 1848 Public Health Act was passed, which allowed any town to set up its own local board of health to tackle public health problems. However, because the 1848 Act was not compulsory very few towns chose to set up health boards or spend money on improving living conditions, so the Act had little impact on improving public health. It wasn't until 1875, more than thirty years after Chadwick's report was published, that the government finally took effective action to tackle public health problems by introducing a compulsory Public Health Act.

2 This question is level marked. You should look at the level descriptions on page 67 to help you mark your answer. Here are some points your answer may include:
- Louis Pasteur's work on the Germ Theory was important because it provided an accurate understanding of the causes of disease. Pasteur's work, which he published in 1861, showed that microbes in the air cause decay, and that some of these microbes cause disease. Before this, most people believed in the miasma theory, which argued that bad air caused disease. By replacing the incorrect miasma theory with the correct Germ Theory, Pasteur enabled people to develop effective ways to treat and prevent disease.
- Pasteur's Germ Theory helped inspire Joseph Lister to develop antiseptics. Lister heard about the Germ Theory in 1865 and realised that germs could be in the air, on surgical instruments and on people's hands. As a result, he started using carbolic acid on instruments and bandages. This was important for the development of medicine because antiseptics allowed surgeons to operate with less fear of patients dying from infection.
- The work of Louis Pasteur was important because it increased understanding about how to prevent disease. For example, Pasteur's work confirmed John Snow's findings about cholera. During a cholera

outbreak in 1853-54, John Snow had shown that there was a connection between contaminated water and cholera. Pasteur's Germ Theory confirmed this link and showed that cleaning towns could help to stop the spread of disease.

- Pasteur's work was important for the development of medicine because Robert Koch was able to build on Pasteur's findings to make his own discoveries about microbes. Koch built on the Germ Theory by linking specific diseases to the particular microbe that caused them. This was important because it allowed other microbe hunters to find the specific bacteria that cause other diseases, and this helped doctors to develop ways of combatting these diseases.

- Pasteur's work was important because he developed vaccines for a number of diseases. After hearing of Koch's discovery of the anthrax bacteria in 1877, Pasteur developed vaccines for anthrax and rabies by testing attenuated cultures on animals such as sheep. As well as providing effective ways of protecting people against these diseases, this work was also important because it developed scientific testing methods.

3 This question is level marked. You should look at the level descriptions on page 67 to help you mark your answer. Here are some points your answer may include:
- In both periods, public health problems were caused by overcrowding in towns and cities. In the Middle Ages, houses in towns were crowded together. This meant that overcrowding and fires were common problems. During the industrial revolution, so many people moved from the countryside to towns to work that good housing couldn't be built quickly enough. This meant that houses were built as close together as possible and overcrowding was a big problem. Workers tried to live in the smallest possible spaces, with whole families often living in a single room.

- In both periods, people didn't fully understand the causes of disease, and this contributed to public health problems. In the Middle Ages, many towns didn't have clean water supplies, so people had to get their drinking water from contaminated rivers and wells, which caused disease. However, people didn't understand the link between dirty water and disease, so there were only limited efforts to solve this problem. A lack of understanding about the causes of disease continued to cause public health problems during the industrial revolution. In this period, water companies set up water pumps in the streets, but their water supply was often contaminated by waste from cesspits or rivers, causing diseases like cholera. This problem wasn't tackled until the second half of the 19th century because people didn't know about the link between cholera and contaminated water until John Snow's work in 1853-54.

- Public health in both periods was affected by a lack of adequate sewerage systems. In the Middle Ages, people in towns would throw their waste into the street or into rivers to be washed away. Sewage from latrines often leaked into the ground and contaminated wells. Similarly, during the industrial revolution, most houses had no bathroom and people shared an outside toilet called a privy. Each privy was built above a cesspit, and nightmen would come to throw waste into rivers or pile it up to be washed away by rain. In London, the lack of an adequate sewerage system led to the 'Great Stink' in 1858.

- In both periods, there were efforts to improve public health by cleaning up towns and cities. For example, in the Middle Ages, York and London both banned people from dumping waste in the street, while London eventually banned any waste from being thrown into the Thames. Many towns ordered toxic businesses, such as butchers, tanners and fishmongers, to move outside the city walls. In the 19th century, measures were also taken to try to improve public health by making towns and cities more hygienic. Between 1859 and 1865, Joseph Bazalgette built a new London sewer system that aimed to get rid of the 'Great Stink' by transporting waste away from heavily populated areas to the Thames Estuary. The 1875 Public Health Act also made towns more hygienic by forcing councils to maintain sewerage systems and keep their towns' streets clean.

4 This question is level marked. You should look at the level descriptions on page 67 to help you mark your answer. Here are some points your answer may include:
- Although there wasn't much progress in surgery in the Middle Ages, individuals played the most important role in the limited development that was achieved. For example, the Italian surgeon Hugh of Lucca and his son Theodoric made several improvements to surgery in the early 13th century. They began dressing wounds with bandages soaked in wine to keep them clean and prevent infection. They also realised that pus was not a healthy sign.

- Individuals continued to play an important role in the development of surgery after the Middle Ages. In the 16th century Ambroise Paré improved the treatment of amputations by developing a method using ligatures, which was less painful than cauterisation and reduced the risk of the patient dying of shock. In the 18th century, John Hunter had a great influence on the development of surgery. Hunter introduced a new approach to the treatment of gunshot wounds, found a new way to treat aneurysms and encouraged good scientific habits such as learning as much about the body as possible to understanding illness and experimenting to find better treatments.

- Individuals had an important influence on the development of anaesthetics and antiseptics in surgery in the late 18th and 19th centuries. A number of doctors and scientists, such as Humphry Davy, Crawford Long and James Simpson, developed new kinds of anaesthetics in this period, including nitrous oxide, ether and chloroform, which helped to solve the problem of pain. In the 1860s, Joseph Lister helped to pioneer the use of carbolic acid as an antiseptic in surgery. This reduced the risk of infection, greatly reducing death rates.

Answers

- In the modern period, new technology has been the most important factor in the development of surgery. For example, advances in laser technology have meant that laser surgery can be used to correct vision problems. Advances in video technology have led to the development of keyhole surgery, which allows the surgeon to see and operate inside the body without making large cuts in the skin. This leaves patients with smaller scars and reduces the risk of infection as a result of surgery.
- Since c.1000, war has been important in the development of surgery. In the 1500s, Ambroise Paré treated many serious injuries caused by war and as a result developed some improved surgical techniques. For example, gunshots wounds often became infected, and he discovered that a cool salve was a better way of preventing this than burning them with a hot iron or pouring boiling oil onto them. In the early 20th century, the First World War contributed to improvements in plastic surgery because Harold Gillies developed the use of pedicle tubes to treat soldiers with facial injuries. His work on plastic surgery was continued during the Second World War by his assistant, Archibald McIndoe, who treated pilots who had been trapped inside burning aircraft.

Modern Medicine

Page 51 — The Impact of the First World War

Knowledge and Understanding

1 a) Wilhelm Röntgen discovered X-rays in 1895.
   b) In 1913, William Coolidge invented the 'Coolidge tube', which was more reliable than the glass tubes that had been used in X-ray equipment until then.
   c) In 1914, Marie Curie developed mobile X-ray units that allowed doctors to transport X-ray equipment. She also worked with French scientist Antoine Béclère to set up training schools which taught doctors how to use X-ray equipment.
2 • The blood of the recipient often clotted.
   • Blood clotted if it was stored outside the body.
3 a) Karl Landsteiner's discovery of blood groups revealed that certain blood groups couldn't be mixed together as the blood would clot. This helped to make transfusions more successful because it enabled doctors to prevent clotting by ensuring that the donor's blood group was the same as the patient's.
   b) The use of sodium citrate made blood transfusions more successful because it stopped blood clotting so that it could be stored. This made it possible to set up blood depots.
4 The development of blood transfusions made surgery safer because transfusions enabled surgeons to replace any blood lost during surgery. This helped to prevent patients dying from blood loss.

5 Harold Gillies improved plastic surgery by developing the use of the pedicle tube. This is a skin graft technique where skin is grown from a healthy part of a patient's body and then used to cover scarring. Gillies also kept detailed records of his achievements which helped other doctors like his assistant, Archibald McIndoe, to continue his work.

Thinking Historically

1 a) The First World War was important for improvements in X-ray equipment. X-ray equipment included glass tubes which were unreliable and often stopped working. During the war, the 'Coolidge tube', a more reliable X-ray tube which had been developed in 1913, became increasingly widely used. The war also made X-rays more accessible. Before the First World War, X-ray machines were often located in hospitals miles away from battlefields, but the war prompted scientists to develop mobile X-ray units which allowed doctors to transport X-ray equipment. In addition, the First World War led to an increase in the number of radiologists who could operate X-ray equipment.
   b) During the First World War, many soldiers died of blood loss as a result of serious wounds from gunshots and explosive shells. Therefore, doctors realised that they needed to be able to store blood safely so that they could quickly give wounded soldiers blood transfusions. As a result, the first ever blood depot was set up at the Battle of Cambrai in 1917.
   c) During the First World War, many men suffered serious facial injuries. This created a need for doctors to develop skin graft techniques so they could reconstruct patients' faces.
2 You can answer either way, as long as you explain your answer. For example:
   War played the most important role in the development of these medical techniques. The large number of serious injuries caused by the First World War created an urgent need for new methods of diagnosis and treatment, and this forced individuals to come up with new ideas. Therefore, the First World War significantly accelerated the development of medical techniques like blood transfusions and plastic surgery.

Page 53 — Penicillin

Knowledge and Understanding

1 Penicillin is an antibiotic. It is important because it is used to treat a range of bacterial infections and its discovery led to the development of other antibiotic treatments.
2 Fleming was looking for a way to prevent septic wounds, which are caused by staphylococcal bacteria. In 1928, he realised that by chance a fungal spore had landed on a culture dish on which he had been growing staphylococci. The mould, Penicillium notatum, had stopped the colonies of staphylococci from growing because it produced a substance that killed bacteria. This substance was given the name penicillin.

Answers

3   No one was willing to fund further research, so Fleming was unable to develop the industrial production of penicillin.

4   Florey and Chain didn't have the resources to produce penicillin in large amounts. Even though their patient had begun to recover during the first clinical trial, Florey and Chain ran out of penicillin and the patient died.

Thinking Historically

1 a) Fleming wanted to find a cure for septic wounds, which are caused by staphylococcal bacteria. This eventually led to his discovery of penicillin.

  b) This meant that penicillin could be purified, which was important as penicillin is a natural product. Florey and Chain were then able to carry out a clinical trial of penicillin.

  c) The US government gave out grants to businesses that manufactured penicillin. By 1943, British businesses were also mass-producing penicillin which meant military medics had sufficient amounts by 1944.

  d) This made penicillin more accessible for general use.

2 a) The Second World War created demand for penicillin because the drug was vital in treating soldiers' wounds. This contributed to the success of penicillin because it led to businesses in the USA and Britain mass-producing the drug so that it could be widely used.

  b) Chance contributed to the success of penicillin because it led to the discovery of the drug in the first place. A spore of Penicillium notatum landed on one of Fleming's culture dishes containing staphylococci by chance, and this led to Fleming's discovery that the fungus produces a substance that kills bacteria.

  c) In December 1941, the US government started giving out grants to businesses that manufactured penicillin. This was important for the success of penicillin because it encouraged US firms to mass-produce the drug. Before this, they had been reluctant to help Florey produce penicillin.

3   You can choose any of the factors, as long as you explain your answer. For example:
    Chance was the most important factor for the success of penicillin. If the fungal spore hadn't landed on one of Fleming's culture dishes, it is unlikely that he would ever have realised that Penicillium notatum could be used to kill bacteria. Therefore he might never have produced penicillin. War and the government were only able to contribute to the success of penicillin because it had been discovered through chance in the first place.

Page 55 — Modern Treatments

Knowledge and Understanding

1   Chemical industries in countries like Britain, Germany, Switzerland and the United States were booming in the late 1800s. This meant chemical companies were able to manufacture newly discovered drugs like aspirin, insulin, sulphonamides and penicillin on a large scale and make them available to a lot of people. The success of their mass-produced drugs in the 1940s helped the modern pharmaceutical industry take off.

2 a) Chemotherapy first began to be developed as a way to treat cancer during the Second World War, and pharmaceutical companies have been producing chemotherapy drugs since the 1960s.

  b) In 1987, pharmaceutical companies began producing AZT. This was the first approved drug to treat the HIV virus, which causes AIDS. Since then they have been involved in developing more effective treatments for HIV.

  c) Pharmaceutical companies produce treatments that reduce the symptoms of SARS, which can include severe breathing difficulties.

3   In the 1950s, the sleeping pill thalidomide was released without thorough testing. It became widely used by pregnant women to treat morning sickness, but this led to thousands of children being born with under-developed limbs and other issues. This tragedy led to improvements in drug safety because the government responded by setting up a Committee on Safety of Drugs in 1963. The committee aimed to make sure all new drugs were safe before being given to patients, so this forced pharmaceutical companies to test drugs more thoroughly.

4   The high costs of researching and developing new medicines mean that pharmaceutical companies tend to focus on treatments for common diseases that will make a lot of money. As a result, treatments for rare diseases sometimes aren't researched because they won't make as much money.

Source Analysis

1 a) The author of the source is the medical director of Public Health England, an important medical organisation. This makes the source useful for studying antibiotic resistance, because the author is likely to have a detailed and informed understanding of the problem.

  b) The source's content is useful because it highlights the severity of the risk posed by antibiotic resistance. Cosford suggests that 'in the not-too distant future' cancer patients and people recovering from surgery might be at risk of 'life-threatening situations' as a result of antibiotic resistance. This reflects the fact that around 25,000 people already die in the European Union every year as a result of infections caused by antibiotic-resistant bacteria.

  c) The purpose of the source is to help tackle antibiotic resistance by persuading the public to only take antibiotics 'when necessary'. This is useful because it gives an insight into the measures that are being taken to tackle the problem of antibiotic resistance. However, the usefulness of the source is limited because it only covers one approach to tackling the problem and it doesn't provide any information about how effective attempts to tackle the problem have been.

Answers

Page 57 — Modern Treatments

Knowledge and Understanding

1 Immunosuppressants are important in organ transplants. They stop the immune system from attacking the implant, which makes organ transplants safer and increases their success rate.

2 a) The discovery of radiation in 1896-1898 by Antoine Henri Becquerel, Marie Curie and Pierre Curie led to the creation of radiation therapy, which involves using radiation to kill cancer cells.

  b) The development of lasers led to their use in many areas of medicine, including cancer treatments and dentistry, as well as laser surgery to correct vision problems.

3 Advances in video technology led to the development of keyhole surgery. This involves putting an endoscope through a small cut so that the surgeon can see inside the body. Other surgical instruments are then introduced through even smaller cuts. Keyhole surgery can be used to investigate the causes of pain and infertility, and for minor operations like vasectomies, removing cysts or the appendix and mending hernias. It leaves patients with smaller scars, reduces the risk of infection and reduces recovery times.

4 • Acupuncture is the method of putting needles into specific points of the patient's skin to relieve pain.
   • Homeopathy is a treatment using extremely weak solutions of natural substances.

5 Alternative treatments aren't based on evidence gathered from scientific research, whereas mainstream treatments are based on experiments and research.

Thinking Historically

1 Surgery in the 19th century:
   • More reliable anaesthetics were developed to solve the problem of pain during surgery.
   • Antiseptics were introduced to kill germs and reduce the risk of infection.
   • Aseptic methods were developed to prevent infection by stopping germs entering the operating theatre.
   Surgery in the 20th century:
   • Doctors worked out how to carry out blood transfusions more successfully, reducing the risk of patients dying from blood loss during surgery.
   • New plastic surgery techniques were developed, such as pedicle tubes, which involve growing skin from a healthy part of a patient's body and using it to cover scarring.
   • Transplants can be carried out successfully. The first successful transplant of the cornea was carried out in 1905, and since then doctors have learnt how to successfully transplant many different organs, including hearts, livers, lungs and kidneys. Increasingly effective immunosuppressants have been developed since the 1970s to make transplant operations safer.
   • Keyhole surgery was developed in the 1980s to allow surgeons to operate through small cuts in the skin. This has made surgery safer, allowing patients to recover more quickly and reducing their risk of infection.

2 You can answer either way, as long as you explain your answer. For example:
   The most important changes to surgery took place during the 19th century. Before this, the problems of pain and infection meant that surgery was very dangerous and only minor procedures could be carried out successfully. It was the development of anaesthetics, antiseptics and aseptic surgery in the 19th century that tackled these problems, massively reducing death rates and making it possible for surgeons to attempt more complex operations. Many of the changes that took place in the 20th century, such as successful organ transplants and developments in plastic surgery, were only possible because of the development of anaesthetics, antiseptics and aseptic surgery in the 19th century.

3 Barber-surgeons:
   • They didn't train at university.
   • They weren't very well respected.
   • As well as carrying out surgery, they also cut hair.
   • They only performed minor operations.
   Modern surgeons:
   • They train at university medical schools.
   • They are highly respected.
   • They carry out a wide variety of complex operations.
   • They have developed many new techniques. In the 20th century these included organ transplants and keyhole surgery.

Page 59 — The Liberal Social Reforms

Thinking Historically

1 a) This report showed that 30% of Londoners were living in severe poverty. Booth found that it was sometimes impossible for people to find work, no matter how hard they tried. His report also showed that even when people did find work, some wages were so low that workers couldn't support their families.

  b) This report showed that severe poverty wasn't just a problem in London. Rowntree showed that 28% of people in York couldn't afford basic food and housing.

2 The reports revealed how widespread and severe poverty was in Britain, and demonstrated that there was often little that poor people could do to help themselves. This may have encouraged the government to become more involved in public health by showing them that poverty and the public health problems it caused needed to be tackled, and that they could only be tackled through government action.

3 When the Boer War broke out in 1899, army officers found that 40% of volunteer soldiers were physically unfit for military service because of poverty-related illnesses linked to poor diet and living conditions. This was important for public health because it showed the government that it needed to improve basic healthcare in order to have an efficient army.

4 a) Children received free schools meals from 1906. From 1907 they were also given free medical inspections at schools.

  b) People over 70 benefited from the old age pensions that were introduced in 1908.

Answers

c) Labour exchanges were introduced in 1909 to help unemployed people find work.

d) Workers benefited from the National Insurance Act that was passed in 1911. It provided health insurance for workers that could be used for sick pay or to pay for a doctor.

Source Analysis

1 The government included David Lloyd George in the image because he was the Chancellor of the Liberal government. They may have shown him sitting next to an ill worker to suggest that the Liberal government cared about workers and wanted to support them.

2 The source creates a positive impression of the Liberal reforms. The title of the leaflet, 'The Dawn of Hope', combined with the reference in the image to 'National Insurance Against Sickness and Disablement', suggests that the government's National Insurance Act will offer workers a brighter future by supporting them if they become unwell.

3 The Liberal government wanted to create a positive impression of their reforms in order to persuade workers to support them. The Liberal reforms represented a major change to the role of the national government in people's lives because they were the first real effort by the government to improve people's living conditions as a way of improving their health. Therefore, the Liberal government may have felt the need to create a positive impression of their reforms in order to persuade people that they were a good idea.

4 The source is limited in its usefulness for an investigation into attitudes towards the Liberal reforms. The source was produced by the Liberal government in order to persuade people to support their reforms, so it doesn't give a balanced view of attitudes towards the reforms. The source presents the reforms in a positive way, but it does not show whether people in Britain shared this positive attitude towards the reforms, or whether some people saw the reforms as something negative.

Page 61 — Public Health and the World Wars

Knowledge and Understanding

1 The government wasn't very successful at tackling the problem of poor-quality housing after the First World War. The Prime Minister, David Lloyd George, promised to build 'homes fit for heroes', and some new council houses were built in the 1920s and 1930s. However, many of the poorest families continued to live in slums because they couldn't afford these new houses.

2 a) During the Second World War, destruction from bombing and a lack of construction led to severe housing shortages.

b) The Labour government built 800,000 new homes.

c) The Labour government passed the New Towns Act which created new towns near major cities.

d) Over 900,000 old, cramped slums were demolished and around 2 million inhabitants were rehoused.

e) A report called 'Homes for Today and Tomorrow' gave specific standards for new housing, including adequate heating, a flushing toilet and enough space inside and outside.

3 The Beveridge Report said that people should have the right to be free from the five 'giants', want, disease, ignorance, squalor and idleness. Beveridge also argued that the government had a duty to care for all citizens, not just the poor or unemployed. Therefore, Beveridge recommended that the state should provide social security 'from the cradle to the grave'. He recommended doing this by creating a welfare state — a system of grants and services available to all British citizens.

4 This Act supported people who couldn't find work, whether as a result of sickness, pregnancy, unemployment or old age. Anyone could apply for National Insurance without having to take a test to see if they were eligible.

5 The 1946 Act was different from the one passed in 1911 because it allowed anyone to apply for National Insurance without having to take a test to see if they were eligible. This may be because the 1946 Act resulted from the Beveridge Report, which said that the government had a duty to care for all its citizens, not just the poor or unemployed.

Thinking Historically

1 First World War:
- Towards the end of the war, David Lloyd George promised to build 'homes fit for heroes'. As a result, the government built some new council houses in the 1920s and 1930s. This only had a limited impact on living conditions because the new houses were too expensive for the poorest families who continued living in slums.
- Raising a mass army to fight the war made the government and military officials more aware of the health problems of the poor because so many recruits were in poor health. The war made the government more concerned with solving these problems because of the need for a strong army to defend the country.

Second World War:
- The evacuation of children increased awareness in richer rural communities of how disadvantaged many people in Britain were. This affected living conditions and public health because it encouraged people to look for improvements in society after the war. Such feelings led to the 1945 victory for the Labour Party, which promised to implement Beveridge's proposals for a welfare state.
- As in the First World War, raising a mass army highlighted health problems among the poor and encouraged the government to tackle them.
- Bombing and a lack of construction during the Second World War led to 800,000 new homes being built by the Labour Government between 1945 and 1951.

Answers

Page 63 — National Health Service

Knowledge and Understanding

1 a) William Beveridge proposed the idea of the National Health Service.

b) Aneurin Bevan was the Labour Minister for Health who introduced the NHS in 1948.

2 • Conservatives opposed the NHS because they believed it would be enormously expensive.

• Doctors opposed the NHS because they saw themselves as independent professionals, so they didn't want to be controlled by the government.

• Some doctors opposed the NHS because they were worried they would lose a lot of income.

3 The Emergency Medical Service was created during the Second World War, and involved the government taking control of all hospitals. It contributed to the creation of the NHS because it was so successful that it persuaded many people to support the idea of the NHS.

4 The NHS has increased the number of people with access to healthcare. It ensures that people have access to a range of vital services, such as accident and emergency care, maternity care, major surgery, pharmacies, dentists, mental health services, sexual health services and GPs. This has contributed to a dramatic rise in life expectancy from 66 years for men and 72 years for women in 1951 to 79 years for men and 83 years for women in 2011.

5 • The increase in life expectancy means that the number of older people in Britain has increased. Older people are more likely to suffer from long-term conditions like diabetes and heart disease, so they need regular medical attention. This requires a lot of NHS time and resources.

• Lifestyle choices put a strain on the NHS. For example, smoking, obesity and alcohol consumption can harm people's health and may require expensive treatment.

• Many modern treatments, equipment and medicines are very expensive.

• The NHS faces rising expectations of what it can and should offer.

• The cost of the NHS is rising rapidly. This means that the NHS sometimes has to make difficult choices about which treatments it can and can't provide in order to stay within its budget.

Thinking Historically

1 a) • At the beginning of the 19th century, most people believed in a laissez-faire style of government, so the government only played a very limited role in public health.

• The government supported Jenner's smallpox vaccination. In 1802, they gave Jenner £10,000 to set up a vaccination clinic, and they gave him a further £20,000 a few years later. They went on to make the vaccination free for infants in 1840 and made it compulsory in 1853. This led to a big fall in the number of smallpox cases in Britain.

• In 1848, the government passed a Public Health Act. This set up a central Board of Health and allowed any town to set up its own local board of health as long as the town's taxpayers agreed. However, this only had a limited impact on public health because few towns chose to set up health boards or spend money improving conditions, and the central health board was dismantled after ten years.

• In 1859, the government responded to the 'Great Stink' by appointing Joseph Bazalgette to build a new London sewer system that would transport waste away from heavily populated areas to the Thames Estuary. This improved public health in London by cleaning up the city's drinking water and ending cholera outbreaks.

• In 1875, the government passed a Public Health Act which forced councils to appoint health inspectors and sanitary inspectors to make sure that laws on things like water supplies and hygiene were followed. It also made councils maintain sewerage systems and keep town streets clean. This Act had a greater impact on public health than the one passed in 1848 because it was compulsory.

• In 1875, the government passed the Artisans' Dwellings Act, which let local councils buy slums with poor living conditions and rebuild them in line with government-backed housing standards. This Act only had a limited impact on public health because few councils chose to use it.

b) • Between 1906 and 1911, the government passed the Liberal reforms, which aimed to improve public health by tackling poverty. The reforms provided support for school children, workers, the unemployed and the elderly.

• After the Second World War, the government improved public health by tackling the problem of poor living conditions. 800,000 new homes were built between 1945 and 1951, and in 1946 the New Towns Act was passed, which created new towns near major cities. Throughout the 1950s and 1960s, the government also demolished over 900,000 old, cramped slums, rehousing around 2 million people.

• The Labour government that was elected in 1945 responded to the Beveridge Report by establishing the welfare state. One of their first acts was to pass the 1946 National Insurance Act, which supported anyone who couldn't work, whether as a result of sickness, pregnancy, unemployment or old age. They went on to create the NHS in 1948, which provides a range of health services, most of which are free and accessible to everyone.

2 You can answer either way, as long as you explain your answer. For example:
The government had a bigger impact on public health in the 20th century because the measures it introduced in this period were more successful and tackled a wider range of problems. Many of the measures introduced by the government in the 19th century,

Answers

such as the 1848 Public Health Act and the 1875 Artisans' Dwellings Act, only had a limited impact on public health. Meanwhile, those measures that were more successful were quite narrow in focus. For example, the government's support for the smallpox vaccination focused on tackling a single disease, while the 1875 Public Health Act focused on a few specific public health issues, such as sewerage and clean water supplies. In contrast, in the 20th century the government tackled a wider range of public health issues, including severe poverty, poor living conditions and access to healthcare. Furthermore, many of the measures introduced by the government during the 20th century have been hugely successful. For example, the NHS contributed to a rise in life expectancy of 13 years for men and 11 years for women between 1951 and 2011.

3   You can choose any of the factors, as long as you explain your answer. For example:
The government was the most important factor in the improvement of public health between c.1880 and c.1960, because it was the driving force behind all the major developments that improved public health in this period, such as the Liberal reforms, the improvements in living conditions after the end of the Second World War and the creation of the NHS. Although the Boer War and the World Wars prompted the government to make some changes, e.g. to living conditions, and William Beveridge played an important role in the creation of the NHS, these changes would have been impossible without government support.

Page 66 — Exam-Style Questions

1   This question is level marked. You should look at the level descriptions on page 67 to help you mark your answer. Here are some points your answer may include:
   • Source A is useful for studying the founding of the NHS because it shows the opposition that Bevan faced from doctors and surgeons. The surgeons at the bottom of the picture are waiting to trip Bevan up and stop him from delivering 'Health for all'. This reflects the fact that many doctors wanted to prevent the foundation of the NHS. Some doctors opposed it because they didn't want to be controlled by the government. They were also worried that the creation of the NHS would cause them to lose a lot of income.
   • This source is useful for studying the founding of the NHS because it gives an insight into public attitudes towards the NHS. In the cartoon, the doctors and surgeons are presented in a negative way. They outnumber Aneurin Bevan and are trying to stop him delivering 'Health for all' by ambushing him with a trip wire. This creates sympathy for Bevan and reflects the fact that despite strong opposition from doctors and Conservatives, the NHS was very popular with the public. Once it had been created, the Conservatives were unable to abolish it when they took power in 1951 because the public liked it so much.

   • The usefulness of the source is limited for an investigation into the founding of the NHS because it was produced in 1945, but the Labour government didn't establish the NHS until 1948. Therefore, although the source reflects doctors' opposition to the NHS before it was created, it doesn't show that the government eventually convinced doctors to back the NHS by offering them a payment for each patient and letting them continue treating fee-paying patients.

2   This question is level marked. You should look at the level descriptions on page 67 to help you mark your answer. Here are some points your answer may include:
   • The huge number of serious injuries from gunshots and explosive shells during the First World War caused many soldiers to die of blood loss. As a result, doctors realised that they needed to be able to store blood so that they could treat blood loss. In 1914, doctors found that sodium citrate stopped blood clotting so it could be stored. This allowed the first blood depot to be set up in 1917, which provided blood for soldiers injured in the Battle of Cambrai. As well as being important for the treatment of serious battle injuries, the ability to store blood was important for the development of surgery because it enabled surgeons to replace any blood lost during an operation, reducing the risk of the patient dying from blood loss.
   • The large number of injuries during the First World War also led to improvements in diagnosis. In 1914, Marie Curie set up mobile X-ray units, allowing X-ray equipment to be transported. The war also led to an increase in the number of radiologists.
   • The First World War was important for improvements in plastic surgery. Harold Gillies set up a plastic surgery unit for the British Army during the war. He used the unit to develop the use of pedicle tubes to complete skin grafts. Gillies' work was continued during the Second World War by Archibald McIndoe.
   • The Second World War was important for the development of penicillin. Penicillin was discovered in 1928 and purified in 1938-40, but mass-production could not begin due to a lack of funding. The US government began funding the mass-production of penicillin in December 1941 after the US entered the war.
   • Both wars led to improvements in living conditions, although the Second World War had a greater impact. Lloyd George promised 'homes fit for heroes' for soldiers returning from the First World War, but the reality failed to live up to his promise. Between 1945 and 1951, 800,000 new homes were built to replace houses destroyed by bombing in the Second World War. These new houses helped to tackle public health problems caused by poor living conditions.
   • The Second World War led to important improvements in public health. The evacuation of children during the war increased the awareness in richer rural communities of how disadvantaged people were elsewhere in the country. After the war, people

looked for ways to improve society, and this led to the election of the Labour government in 1945, who promised to implement the Beveridge Report. In 1948, they introduced the NHS, which had a huge impact on public health because it made health services free for all patients.

3   This question is level marked. You should look at the level descriptions on page 67 to help you mark your answer. Here are some points your answer may include:

- In the Middle Ages, medicines and remedies weren't mass produced, but were often made by apothecaries and local wise women or made at home. The recipes were either passed down or written in books. In contrast, since the end of the 19th century, medicines in Britain have been mass-produced by pharmaceutical companies, which research and develop new drugs. These medicines go through a series of clinical tests to check they're safe. In 1963, the government set up a Committee on Safety of Drugs to make sure this happened.

- Many treatments in the Middle Ages were based on religion or superstition, and there were few advances in medical technology. Many people believed that disease was a punishment from God, so they prayed to saints in the hope they would intervene and stop the illness or made pilgrimages to holy shrines in the belief that this could cure them. In modern Britain, religion plays a less important role in treatment, and treatments are often based on advances in technology and research. For example, modern treatments for cancer often rely on new discoveries and inventions that have been developed in the 20th and 21st centuries, such as radiation, chemotherapy drugs and lasers.

- The methods used to treat disease since c.1900 are much more effective than the treatments that were used in the Middle Ages. In the Middle Ages, treatments were based on incorrect ideas about the causes of disease, so they were usually ineffective. For example, bloodletting and purging were used as treatments because it was believed that they helped to balance the humours. However, bloodletting caused more deaths than it prevented because some people were accidentally killed when too much blood was taken. In contrast, modern treatments for disease are based on a more accurate understanding of the causes of disease and so they are often much safer and more effective. For example, since the 1860s, doctors have known that some bacteria cause disease. In the 20th century, the Germ Theory enabled Fleming, Florey and Chain to develop penicillin, which is used to treat a range of bacterial infections, including chest and skin infections.

- The government has been much more involved in organising and funding the treatment of disease since c.1900 than it was in the Middle Ages. In the Middle Ages, the government had little involvement in healthcare and most people saw an apothecary or a barber-surgeon, unless they could afford to see a physician. In contrast, since c.1900 the government has been heavily involved in making sure that patients receive effective treatments. For example, in 1911 the Liberal government introduced health insurance for workers to pay for a doctor. In 1948, the Labour government set up the NHS, which greatly increased access to healthcare and meant that the government supported a range of treatments, including accident and emergency care and major surgery.

4   This question is level marked. You should look at the level descriptions on page 67 to help you mark your answer. Here are some points your answer may include:

- In the 19th century, the government played the most important role in improving public health. The 1875 Public Health Act was the first compulsory government intervention in public health and was effective in improving towns' water and sewerage systems. The government also supported major projects to improve public health like Bazalgette's sewer system in London and the clearance of Birmingham's slums.

- In the 19th and 20th centuries, the government played an important role in preventing disease. In 1802, Parliament supported Jenner's smallpox vaccine with a £10,000 grant, and in 1853 the government made the vaccination compulsory. In the early 20th century, the Liberal government introduced reforms such as free school meals in 1906 and labour exchanges in 1909 to improve health by tackling poverty.

- In the 20th century, the government played the most important role in improving public health, as it significantly improved access to medical treatment. In 1948, the government established the National Health Service, which has improved people's health by offering a range of medical services free of charge. Furthermore, government action since the Second World War has led to the clearance of slum housing and the improvement of living conditions.

- Other factors were more important in improving public health before the 19th century, as the government believed in a laissez-faire approach towards public health before this time. For example, in the Middle Ages, local and national governments only took limited action to improve living conditions in towns, and there was no national government response to serious epidemics such as the Black Death in the 14th century and the Great Plague in the 17th century. The government's laissez-faire approach did not begin to change until the government granted funding to Jenner's smallpox vaccination clinic in the early 19th century.

Answers

- During the medieval period, the Church was more important than the government in improving people's health, as monasteries ran most hospitals and tried to provide care for the poor, sick and elderly. However, the role of the Church in improving people's health decreased after the 1530s when Henry VIII began the dissolution of the monasteries. This led to the closure of a large number of hospitals, and so reduced the Church's role in improving public health.
- From the 1500s onwards, institutions such as the College of Physicians and the London College of Surgeons played an important role in improving public health because they helped to improve the standard of medical treatment people received. For example, after the College of Physicians was set up in 1518 it issued licences to doctors who had trained at the college. This separated them from quack doctors and helped to stop quackery, which was important for public health because quacks sold medicines that didn't work and often did more harm than good. Similarly, the London College of Surgeons helped to improve standards in surgery by setting training standards for surgeons from 1800 onwards.
- In many cases, government action to improve people's health only came about because of advances in science and technology. For example, from 1861 the growing acceptance of Pasteur's Germ Theory meant that the link between poor living conditions and poor health became more obvious. This provided the scientific proof required to persuade the government to pass the 1875 Public Health Act.

Index